SIMPLE DASH DIET COOKBOOK FOR BEGINNERS

Mouthwatering And Tasty Recipes to Reduce Blood Pressure And Shed Pounds

BY

Hampton Ellison

Copyright © 2024 by [Hampton Ellison]

TABLE OF CONTENTS

INTRODUCTION

Imagine waking up one day, realizing that the relentless pounding in your temples and the constant fatigue aren't just nuisances but alarms from your body signaling something deeper. For Lisa, a 45-year-old mother of two, this realization came abruptly during a routine check-up. Her doctor mentioned a term that was foreign yet ominous: hypertension. With her busy schedule juggling work, kids, and home, Lisa barely had time to think about herself, let alone her diet.

Lisa isn't alone. Millions of people around the world are caught in the whirlwind of modern life, often overlooking their health until it's nearly too late. The statistics are alarming – high blood pressure, heart disease, and related complications are becoming all too common. But there's hope, and it starts with a simple shift in what we eat.

Enter the DASH diet. Developed by nutrition experts to combat hypertension and promote heart health, the DASH (Dietary Approaches to Stop Hypertension) diet has been praised for its effectiveness and simplicity. Unlike fad diets that promise quick fixes, the DASH diet is a sustainable lifestyle change, emphasizing whole foods, balanced nutrition, and delicious meals.

For Lisa, adopting the DASH diet was a game-changer. She found that by making small, manageable changes to her eating habits, she could significantly improve her health without sacrificing flavor or spending hours in the kitchen. The DASH diet became not just a dietary plan but a pathway to reclaiming her vitality and well-being.

This cookbook is designed with beginners like Lisa in mind – those who are new to the DASH diet and may feel overwhelmed by where to start. It's a comprehensive guide, breaking down the principles of the diet into easy-to-understand steps and providing a variety of mouth-watering recipes that are both nutritious and straightforward to prepare.

As you embark on this journey, remember that every small step you take towards healthier eating is a victory. This cookbook is your companion, offering guidance, support, and inspiration. Just as Lisa transformed her health and life with the DASH diet, you too can experience the benefits of eating well.

CHAPTER ONE

What is the DASH Diet?

The DASH diet, short for Dietary Approaches to Stop Hypertension, is a scientifically researched and well-regarded dietary plan designed primarily to combat high blood pressure (hypertension). Developed in the 1990s by the National Heart, Lung, and Blood Institute (NHLBI), the DASH diet has consistently ranked as one of the healthiest diets by nutrition experts and health organizations worldwide. The DASH diet was created through rigorous clinical trials aimed at discovering effective non-pharmacological methods to lower blood pressure. Researchers found that a diet rich in fruits, vegetables, whole grains, and low-fat dairy products, and low in saturated fat, cholesterol, and sodium, significantly reduced blood pressure levels in participants. The DASH diet's success in these trials led to its endorsement by major health organizations such as the American Heart Association and the Dietary Guidelines for Americans.

Core Principles of the DASH Diet

1. **High in Nutrients**: The DASH diet emphasizes the intake of nutrients known to help lower blood pressure, such as potassium, calcium, magnesium,

fiber, and protein. These nutrients are abundant in fruits, vegetables, whole grains, and dairy products.

2. **Low in Sodium**: Reducing sodium intake is a cornerstone of the DASH diet. The standard DASH diet recommends limiting sodium to 2,300 milligrams per day, roughly the amount in one teaspoon of table salt. For those with more significant hypertension or who want to reduce blood pressure even further, a lower sodium version of the diet caps sodium intake at 1,500 milligrams per day.

3. **Rich in Whole Foods**: Processed and packaged foods are often high in sodium and unhealthy fats. The DASH diet encourages the consumption of whole foods, which are less processed and closer to their natural state, providing more nutrients and fewer unhealthy additives.

4. **Balanced and Moderate in Fats**: While the DASH diet does not eliminate fats, it emphasizes healthy fats found in nuts, seeds, and fish, while limiting saturated fats and cholesterol present in fried foods, high-fat dairy products, and fatty meats.

5. **Emphasis on Portion Control**: The DASH diet promotes mindful eating and portion control to avoid overeating, which can contribute to weight gain and higher blood pressure.

Benefits of the DASH Diet

1. **Lower Blood Pressure**: The primary benefit of the DASH diet is its ability to lower blood pressure. Studies have shown that following the DASH diet can reduce systolic blood pressure (the top number in a blood pressure reading) by 8-14 points, which can significantly reduce the risk of heart disease and stroke.

2. **Heart Health**: By reducing blood pressure and lowering cholesterol levels, the DASH diet helps to protect against heart disease. The diet's emphasis on fruits, vegetables, and whole grains also supports overall cardiovascular health.

3. **Weight Management**: The DASH diet is naturally low in calories and high in fiber, which can help with weight loss and maintaining a healthy weight. This is particularly beneficial as obesity is a major risk factor for hypertension.

4. **Reduced Risk of Diabetes**: The diet's focus on whole grains and high-fiber foods can help regulate blood sugar levels and improve insulin sensitivity, reducing the risk of type 2 diabetes.

5. **Overall Nutritional Improvement**: Following the DASH diet can lead to a more balanced and nutrient-rich diet, improving overall health and wellbeing. It encourages the consumption of a wide

variety of foods that provide essential vitamins and minerals.

The DASH diet is more than just a method for lowering blood pressure; it's a comprehensive approach to healthier eating that can benefit your overall health. By focusing on nutrient-rich whole foods and reducing sodium intake, the DASH diet offers a sustainable way to improve your diet and lifestyle. Whether you're looking to lower your blood pressure, manage your weight, or simply adopt healthier eating habits, the DASH diet provides a practical and effective framework for achieving your health goals.

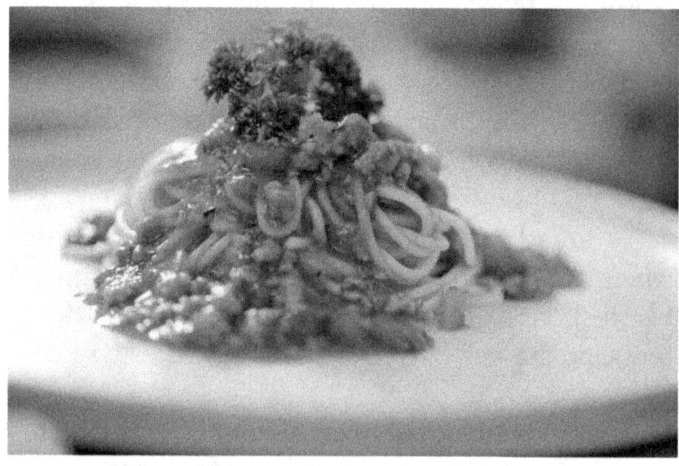

CHAPTER TWO

The Science Behind the DASH Diet

The DASH diet, short for Dietary Approaches to Stop Hypertension, is grounded in a robust body of scientific research aimed at reducing high blood pressure and improving overall cardiovascular health. Developed through rigorous clinical trials and studies funded by the National Institutes of Health (NIH), the DASH diet has become a benchmark in dietary recommendations for those seeking to manage hypertension and related health conditions. This section delves into the scientific principles that underpin the DASH diet and explains why it is effective.

Clinical Trials and Research Foundations

The DASH diet was formulated based on findings from the DASH (Dietary Approaches to Stop Hypertension) clinical trial, which sought to investigate the impact of dietary patterns on blood pressure. This landmark study involved 459 adults with varying levels of hypertension who were randomly assigned to one of three diets: a typical American diet, a diet rich in fruits and vegetables, and the DASH diet.

The results were striking. Participants on the DASH diet experienced significant reductions in both systolic and diastolic blood pressure compared to those on the other two diets. These improvements were observed in both hypertensive and non-hypertensive individuals, highlighting the diet's broad applicability.

Key Nutritional Components

1. **Potassium**:
Potassium is a vital mineral that helps balance sodium levels in the body and relaxes blood vessel walls, which can reduce blood pressure. The DASH diet emphasizes potassium-rich foods such as bananas, oranges, potatoes, and spinach.

2. **Calcium**:
Calcium is essential for maintaining healthy blood pressure. Dairy products, a key component of the DASH diet, are rich in calcium, and the diet includes low-fat or fat-free options to maximize this benefit without increasing fat intake.

3. **Magnesium**: By relaxing blood arteries, magnesium aids in blood pressure regulation. The DASH diet includes magnesium-rich foods like nuts, seeds, whole grains, and leafy green vegetables.

4. **Fiber**: High-fiber foods, such as fruits, vegetables, and whole grains, are staples of the DASH diet. Fiber helps improve overall heart health by lowering cholesterol levels and aiding in weight management.

5. **Low Sodium**: One of the most critical aspects of the DASH diet is its low sodium content. Excess sodium can lead to water retention, which increases blood pressure. The DASH diet recommends limiting sodium intake to 2,300 milligrams per day, with an even stricter limit of 1,500 milligrams for those who need it.

Mechanisms of Action

The DASH diet's effectiveness in lowering blood pressure and promoting heart health can be attributed to several physiological mechanisms:

1. **Electrolyte Balance**: The balance between sodium, potassium, and magnesium is crucial for maintaining healthy blood pressure levels. By increasing potassium and magnesium intake while reducing sodium, the DASH diet helps optimize this balance, leading to lower blood pressure.

2. **Vascular Health**: The nutrients emphasized in the DASH diet, particularly potassium, calcium, and magnesium, contribute to the relaxation and dilation of blood vessels. This helps reduce vascular resistance and lower blood pressure.

3. **Reduced Inflammation**: The DASH diet is rich in antioxidants and anti-inflammatory foods, such as fruits, vegetables, and nuts. These foods help reduce oxidative stress and inflammation, which are linked to hypertension and cardiovascular disease.

4. **Improved Lipid Profile**: The DASH diet's emphasis on whole grains, lean proteins, and healthy fats helps improve cholesterol levels by reducing LDL (bad) cholesterol and increasing HDL (good) cholesterol. A healthier lipid profile reduces the risk of atherosclerosis, a condition characterized by the buildup of plaque in the arteries that can lead to heart attacks and strokes.

5. **Weight Management**: By focusing on nutrient-dense, low-calorie foods, the DASH diet can help with weight loss and weight management. Maintaining a healthy weight is a crucial factor in controlling blood pressure.

Supporting Studies and Long-Term Benefits

Several studies have supported the initial findings of the DASH clinical trial, reinforcing the diet's benefits:

- DASH-Sodium Study: This follow-up study examined the effects of different sodium levels within the context of the DASH diet. It confirmed that reducing sodium intake further lowers blood pressure, even beyond the benefits of the standard DASH diet.

- Meta-Analyses: Numerous meta-analyses have reviewed multiple studies on the DASH diet, consistently finding significant reductions in blood pressure, improved cholesterol levels, and decreased risk of cardiovascular events among those following the diet.

- Diabetes Prevention: Research has shown that the DASH diet can improve insulin sensitivity and reduce the risk of developing type 2 diabetes, further enhancing its role in promoting overall health.

Practical Applications and Broader Impact

The principles of the DASH diet extend beyond individual health benefits and have broader implications for public health:

1. **Public Health Guidelines**: The DASH diet is often incorporated into national dietary guidelines and recommendations, such as the Dietary Guidelines for Americans, due to its proven effectiveness and ease of adoption.

2. **Healthcare Practice**: Healthcare providers frequently recommend the DASH diet to patients with hypertension, prehypertension, and other cardiovascular risk factors as a first-line intervention before or alongside medication.

3. **Community Programs**: Public health initiatives and community programs aimed at reducing hypertension often use the DASH diet as a foundational component, demonstrating its practicality and scalability.

The DASH diet is a scientifically validated approach to improving cardiovascular health through dietary changes. Its emphasis on whole foods rich in potassium, calcium, magnesium, and fiber, combined with reduced sodium intake, creates a balanced and effective strategy for lowering blood pressure and reducing the risk of chronic diseases. The robust body of research supporting the DASH diet underscores its value as a cornerstone of dietary recommendations for individuals and public health initiatives alike.

CHAPTER THREE

Health Benefits of the DASH Diet

The DASH diet, or Dietary Approaches to Stop Hypertension, has been extensively researched and recommended by health professionals worldwide for its numerous health benefits. This eating plan is not only effective in lowering blood pressure but also offers a wide range of other health advantages.

1.Reduction of Blood Pressure

The primary goal of the DASH diet is to lower blood pressure, and it is remarkably effective in achieving this. One of the main risk factors for heart disease, stroke, and kidney disease is high blood pressure, or hypertension. The DASH diet lowers blood pressure by promoting the consumption of nutrients such as potassium, calcium, and magnesium, which help balance sodium levels in the body and support healthy blood vessel function.

- Systolic and Diastolic Pressure: Studies have shown that the DASH diet can reduce systolic blood pressure (the top number) by an average of 8-14 mm Hg and diastolic blood pressure (the bottom number) by 4-10 mm Hg. These reductions are comparable to those achieved with medication, making the DASH diet an excellent first-line intervention for hypertension.

2. Improved Heart Health

By lowering blood pressure, the DASH diet directly contributes to improved heart health. However, its benefits extend beyond just blood pressure reduction:

- Cholesterol Levels: The DASH diet is low in saturated fats and cholesterol, which helps reduce levels of LDL (bad) cholesterol. High LDL cholesterol is a major risk factor for atherosclerosis (the buildup of plaques in the arteries), which can lead to heart attacks and strokes. The diet also promotes the intake of healthy fats, which can help raise HDL (good) cholesterol levels.

- Heart Disease Risk: By improving blood pressure and cholesterol levels, the DASH diet significantly reduces the risk of developing heart disease. Research has shown that people who follow the DASH diet have a lower incidence of coronary heart disease and other cardiovascular conditions.

3. Weight Management and Obesity Prevention

The DASH diet is naturally low in calories and high in fiber, which can aid in weight loss and weight management:

- Satiety: Foods emphasized in the DASH diet, such as fruits, vegetables, and whole grains, are high in fiber and promote a feeling of fullness. This helps reduce overall calorie intake without the need for restrictive dieting.

- Sustainable Eating Patterns: The DASH diet encourages balanced meals with appropriate portion sizes, making it easier to maintain a healthy weight over the long term.

4. **Reduced Risk of Diabetes**

The DASH diet's focus on whole grains, lean proteins, and high-fiber foods can help regulate blood sugar levels and improve insulin sensitivity:

- Type 2 Diabetes: Studies have shown that individuals following the DASH diet have a lower risk of developing type 2 diabetes. The diet helps manage blood glucose levels and reduces the likelihood of insulin resistance.

- Glycemic Control: For those with diabetes, the DASH diet can improve glycemic control and reduce the need for medication by promoting foods with a low glycemic index.

5. **Prevention and Management of Metabolic Syndrome**

A group of illnesses known as metabolic syndrome raise the risk of diabetes, heart disease, and stroke. High blood pressure, high blood sugar, excess body fat around the waist, and abnormal cholesterol levels are some of these problems. The DASH diet can help manage and prevent metabolic syndrome by addressing each of these components:

- Blood Pressure and Cholesterol: As discussed, the DASH diet is effective in lowering blood pressure and improving cholesterol levels.
- Blood Sugar Control: The diet's emphasis on whole foods and balanced meals helps maintain stable blood sugar levels.
- Weight Management: By promoting a healthy weight, the DASH diet reduces abdominal fat, a key factor in metabolic syndrome.

6. **Improved Kidney Function**

Diabetes and high blood pressure are the main risk factors for chronic renal disease. By managing these conditions, the DASH diet helps protect kidney function:

- Reduced Proteinuria: The DASH diet has been shown to reduce proteinuria (excess protein in the urine), which is a marker of kidney damage.

- Slowed Progression of Kidney Disease: For individuals with existing kidney disease, the DASH diet can help slow the progression by managing blood pressure and blood sugar levels.

7. Enhanced Bone Health

The DASH diet's emphasis on calcium-rich foods, such as low-fat dairy products, supports bone health. Adequate calcium intake is essential for maintaining strong bones and preventing osteoporosis, particularly in older adults.

8. Cancer Prevention

There is emerging evidence that the DASH diet may help reduce the risk of certain cancers. The diet's high intake of fruits and vegetables provides a wealth of antioxidants and phytochemicals, which have been linked to lower rates of cancer:

- Colorectal Cancer: Some studies have suggested that the DASH diet is associated with a reduced risk of colorectal cancer due to its high fiber content and the presence of protective nutrients found in fruits and vegetables.
- Breast Cancer: There is also evidence to suggest that following the DASH diet can lower the risk of breast cancer, possibly due to its overall healthy eating pattern and weight management benefits.

9. **Improved Mental Health**

Emerging research indicates that diet can play a crucial role in mental health. The DASH diet's nutrient-rich foods, particularly those high in antioxidants, omega-3 fatty acids, and vitamins, can support brain health and cognitive function:

- Cognitive Decline: Some studies have linked the DASH diet with a reduced risk of cognitive decline and dementia. The diet's emphasis on whole foods and healthy fats is thought to support brain health and reduce inflammation.
- Mood Disorders: A balanced diet like the DASH diet can help stabilize mood and reduce the risk of depression. Nutrients such as omega-3 fatty acids, found in fish and nuts, are particularly beneficial for mental health.

10. **Overall Nutritional Improvement**

The DASH diet promotes a well-rounded, balanced diet that provides essential nutrients for overall health and well-being:

- Micronutrients: By encouraging the consumption of a variety of fruits, vegetables, whole grains, and lean proteins, the DASH diet ensures adequate intake of essential vitamins and minerals.
- Antioxidants: The high intake of fruits and vegetables provides a rich source of antioxidants, which help protect the body from oxidative stress and inflammation.

The DASH diet offers a comprehensive approach to health that goes beyond just lowering blood pressure. It also provides a wide range of health benefits, from improved heart health and weight management to reduced risk of diabetes, cancer prevention, and enhanced mental well-being.

DASH Diet Guidelines and Nutritional Goals

The DASH (Dietary Approaches to Stop Hypertension) diet is a well-structured eating plan designed to promote cardiovascular health and prevent high blood pressure. This diet emphasizes the consumption of nutrient-rich foods while limiting those that can negatively impact health. Here is a comprehensive overview of the guidelines and nutritional goals of the DASH diet.

1. **Emphasize Fruits and Vegetables**: Fruits and vegetables are the foundation of the DASH diet. They are rich in essential vitamins, minerals, fiber, and antioxidants that support overall health and help manage blood pressure.

2. **Choose Whole Grains**: Whole grains are preferred over refined grains due to their higher fiber content and nutrient density. Whole wheat, brown rice, quinoa, barley, and oats are a few examples.

3. **Include Low-Fat Dairy**: Low-fat or fat-free dairy products are important for providing calcium, vitamin D, and protein without the added saturated fat found in full-fat dairy products.

4. **Opt for Lean Proteins**: Lean sources of protein, such as poultry, fish, beans, and legumes, are emphasized. Red meat should be limited, and processed meats should be avoided.

5. **Healthy Fats**: Healthy fats, particularly those from nuts, seeds, and fish, are encouraged. Saturated and trans fats should be minimized.

6. **Limit Sodium Intake**: Reducing sodium intake is a key aspect of the DASH diet. This involves avoiding highly processed foods and being mindful of added salt in home-cooked meals.

7. **Moderate Sweets and Sugars**: Foods and beverages high in added sugars should be limited to occasional treats.

Daily and Weekly Serving Recommendations

The DASH diet provides specific guidelines on the number of servings from each food group to help achieve its nutritional goals. Serving sizes and recommendations can vary based on individual calorie needs, but a standard 2,000-calorie per day DASH diet typically includes:

1. **Grains**: 6-8 Servings per Day
   - Examples: 1 slice of whole wheat bread, 1 ounce of dry cereal, 1/2 cup of cooked rice, pasta, or cereal.
   - Nutritional Goal: Provide energy, fiber, and essential nutrients like B vitamins.

2. **Vegetables**: 4-5 Servings per Day
   - Examples: 1 cup of raw leafy vegetables, 1/2 cup of cooked vegetables, 1/2 cup of vegetable juice.
   - Nutritional Goal: Supply vitamins, minerals (such as potassium and magnesium), and fiber.

3. **Fruits**: 4-5 Servings per Day
   - Examples: 1 medium fruit, 1/2 cup of fresh, frozen, or canned fruit, 1/2 cup of fruit juice.
   - Nutritional Goal: Provide essential vitamins (like vitamin C), minerals, and fiber.

4. **Dairy**: 2-3 Servings per Day
   - Examples: 1 cup of milk or yogurt, 1.5 ounces of cheese.
   - Nutritional Goal: Deliver calcium, vitamin D, and protein.

5. **Lean Meats, Poultry, and Fish**: 6 or Fewer Servings per Day
   - Examples: 1 ounce of cooked meat, poultry, or fish, 1 egg.

- Nutritional Goal: Provide protein, B vitamins, iron, and zinc.

6. **Legumes**, Nuts, and Seeds: 4-5 Servings Weekly
   - Examples: 1/3 cup of nuts, 2 tablespoons of seeds, 1/2 cup of cooked beans or peas.
   - Nutritional Goal: Supply protein, magnesium, potassium, fiber, and healthy fats.

7. **Fats and Oils**: 2-3 Servings per Day
   - Examples: 1 teaspoon of soft margarine, 1 tablespoon of mayonnaise, 2 tablespoons of salad dressing.
   - Nutritional Goal: Provide essential fatty acids and fat-soluble vitamins while keeping saturated fat low.

8. **Sweets and Added Sugars**: 5 or Fewer Servings per Week
   - Examples: 1 tablespoon of sugar, jelly, or jam, 1/2 cup of sorbet, 1 cup of lemonade.
   - Nutritional Goal: Minimize intake of empty calories and excessive sugar.

Nutritional Goals of the DASH Diet

The DASH diet is designed to achieve several key nutritional goals that contribute to overall health and the management of blood pressure.

1. **High Potassium**: Aim for about 4,700 mg per day. Potassium helps balance sodium levels and reduces tension in blood vessel walls, which lowers blood pressure.

2. **High Calcium**: Aim for 1,000-1,300 mg per day. Calcium is crucial for maintaining strong bones and plays a role in vascular contraction and vasodilation.

3. **High Magnesium**: Aim for 420 mg per day for men and 320 mg per day for women. Magnesium promotes healthy blood pressure regulation as well as neuron and muscle function.

4. **Adequate Fiber**: Aim for 25-30 grams per day. Fiber helps reduce cholesterol levels, control blood sugar, and promote healthy digestion.

5. **Low Sodium**: Standard DASH diet recommends less than 2,300 mg per day, with an optimal target of 1,500 mg per day for individuals with hypertension or those looking to maximize blood pressure reduction.

6. **Healthy Fats**: Focus on monounsaturated and polyunsaturated fats while limiting saturated and trans fats. This balance supports heart health and helps manage cholesterol levels.

7. **Controlled Caloric Intake**: Adhering to calorie needs based on age, sex, and activity level helps

maintain a healthy weight, which is crucial for blood pressure control and overall health.

Practical Tips for Following the DASH Diet

1. **Gradual Transition**: Start by making small changes, such as adding an extra serving of vegetables or choosing whole grain bread instead of white bread.

2. **Read Labels**: Pay attention to nutrition labels to monitor sodium, sugar, and fat content.

3. **Plan Meals**: Plan your meals ahead of time to ensure a balanced diet and avoid last-minute unhealthy choices.

4. **Cook at Home**: Preparing meals at home allows you to control ingredients and make healthier choices.

5. **Portion Control**: Be mindful of portion sizes to avoid overeating, especially with high-calorie foods.

6. **Stay Hydrated**: Drink plenty of water throughout the day and limit sugary drinks and alcohol.

7. **Incorporate Variety**: Include a wide range of foods from all the food groups to ensure a balanced intake of nutrients.

CHAPTER FOUR

Setting Realistic Goals

Embarking on the DASH (Dietary Approaches to Stop Hypertension) diet is a positive step towards better health and well-being. However, the success of any dietary change relies heavily on setting realistic and achievable goals. Setting realistic goals can help you stay motivated and on track.

Importance of Realistic Goals

Setting realistic goals is crucial because:

1. **Sustainability**: Achievable goals are more likely to be sustained over the long term. Unrealistic goals can lead to frustration and burnout, making it harder to stick with the diet.

2. **Motivation**: Realistic goals provide a clear path to success and a sense of accomplishment, which can boost motivation and confidence.

3. **Measurable Progress**: Specific and attainable goals allow you to track progress more effectively, helping you to see the tangible benefits of your efforts.

Steps to Setting Realistic Goals

1. Assess Your Starting Point
   - Health Assessment: Begin by assessing your current health status. This might involve measuring your blood pressure, weight, and cholesterol levels. Understanding your starting point can help you set appropriate targets and track your progress.
   - Dietary Habits: Evaluate your current eating habits. Identify areas where you can make improvements, such as reducing sodium intake or increasing the consumption of fruits and vegetables.

2. Set Specific Goals
   - Be Specific: Instead of setting vague goals like "eat healthier," aim for specific targets such as "eat at least five servings of vegetables daily" or "reduce sodium intake to 1,500 mg per day."
   - Quantify Your Goals: Use numbers to make your goals measurable. For instance, "exercise for 30 minutes, five days a week" and "drink eight glasses of water daily."

3. Make Goals Attainable
   - Start Small: Begin with small, manageable changes. For instance, if you currently eat one serving of vegetables a day, aim to increase it to two servings before gradually increasing further.

  - Build on Success: Once you achieve smaller goals, set new ones that build on your success. This step-by-step approach can help maintain momentum and prevent feeling overwhelmed.

4. Set Relevant Goals
  - Align with Health Needs: Ensure your goals are relevant to your health needs. For example, if you have high blood pressure, focus on goals that help lower it, such as reducing sodium intake and increasing potassium-rich foods.
  - Personal Relevance: Choose goals that resonate with your personal values and lifestyle. If you enjoy cooking, a goal like "prepare three new DASH-friendly recipes each week" may be more engaging.

5. Establish a Timeline
  - Short-Term Goals: Set short-term goals that can be achieved within a few weeks. These provide quick wins and keep you motivated. For example, "reduce soda consumption by half within the next month."
  - Long-Term Goals: Set long-term goals that span several months to a year. These should align with your overall health objectives, such as "reach and maintain a healthy blood pressure level within six months."

6. **Monitor and Adjust Goals**
   - Track Progress: Continually assess how well you're doing in reaching your objectives. Use a journal, app, or calendar to record your achievements and any challenges you encounter.
   - Be Flexible: Be ready to modify your objectives as necessary. If a goal proves too difficult or too easy, modify it to better suit your needs and circumstances.

Examples of Realistic Goals for the DASH Diet

1. Dietary Goals
   - Increase Vegetable Intake: "Eat at least four servings of vegetables each day for the next month."
   - Reduce Sodium Intake: "Limit daily sodium intake to 2,300 mg for the next two weeks, then reduce to 1,500 mg over the following month."
   - Choose Whole Grains: "Replace white bread and pasta with whole grain alternatives within the next two weeks."

2. Lifestyle Goals
   - Physical Activity: "Walk briskly for 30 minutes, five days a week, for the next month."
   - Hydration: "Drink eight glasses of water each day for the next month."

3. **Behavioral Goals**
   - "Mental Eating": "Practice mindful eating by
savoring each bite and eating without distractions
at least once a day."
   - Meal Planning: "Plan and prepare a week's
worth of DASH-friendly meals every Sunday for the
next month."

Tips for Achieving Your Goals

1. **Create a Support System**
   - Family and Friends: Involve family and friends in
your journey. Their help can provide motivation and
accountability.
   - Join a Community: Consider joining a support
group or online community focused on the DASH
diet or healthy eating. It can inspire others to
provide advice and experiences.

2. **Educate Yourself**
   - Learn About Nutrition: Invest time in learning
about nutrition and the principles of the DASH diet.
Understanding why certain foods are beneficial can
reinforce healthy choices.
   - Explore Recipes: Experiment with
DASH-friendly recipes to keep your meals
enjoyable and varied.

3. **Prepare for Challenges**
   - Identify Triggers: Recognize situations or
emotions that may trigger unhealthy eating habits.

Create coping mechanisms to handle these stressors.

- Plan for Setbacks: Accept that setbacks are part of the journey. Instead of being discouraged, use them as learning opportunities and adjust your approach as needed.

4. **Celebrate Successes**

-Recognize Progress: Take pride in your accomplishments, no matter how tiny. Recognizing your progress can boost motivation and reinforce positive behavior.

- Reward Yourself: Reward yourself for meeting your goals. Choose non-food rewards, such as a new book, a relaxing bath, or a fun activity.

Setting realistic goals is a fundamental step in successfully adopting and maintaining the DASH diet. By assessing your starting point, setting specific, attainable, and relevant goals, establishing a timeline, and monitoring your progress, you can create a sustainable path to better health. Recall that adopting a healthy lifestyle is a marathon, not a sprint. Over time, minor adjustments made on a regular basis might provide major gains. Embrace the process, stay flexible, and celebrate your successes along the way.

CHAPTER FIVE

Kitchen Essentials: Must-Have Tools and Gadgets

Embarking on the DASH diet involves more than just choosing the right foods; it also means equipping your kitchen with the right tools and gadgets to make meal preparation efficient, enjoyable, and successful.

Basic Cooking Utensils

1. **Knives**
   - Chef's Knife: A versatile knife essential for chopping vegetables, slicing fruits, and cutting meats. Invest in a high-quality, sharp chef's knife to make food preparation easier and safer.
   - Paring Knife: Ideal for peeling and intricate tasks like de-seeding fruits and vegetables.
   - Bread Knife: A serrated knife perfect for slicing bread and other baked goods.

2. **Cutting Boards**
   - Wooden or Bamboo: Great for vegetables and fruits.
   - Plastic or Non-Porous: Essential for cutting raw meat to prevent cross-contamination. Consider color-coded boards to avoid mixing up.

3. **Measuring Tools**

- Measuring Cups: Both liquid and dry measuring cups are necessary for accurate portion control and recipe success.
- Measuring Spoons: For measuring small amounts of ingredients like spices, baking powder, or oil.

4. **Mixing Bowls**

- Variety of Sizes: Stainless steel or glass bowls in various sizes for mixing salads, doughs, and batters.

5. **Wooden Spoons and Spatulas**

- Wooden Spoons: Ideal for stirring and mixing without scratching your cookware.
- Silicone Spatulas: Heat-resistant and perfect for scraping bowls and pans.

Cookware and Bakeware

1. **Pots and Pans**

- Non-Stick Skillet: For sautéing vegetables and cooking lean proteins with minimal oil.
- Cast Iron Skillet: Adaptable and excellent for cooking at high temperatures.
- Saucepan: For making sauces, boiling grains, and cooking soups.
- Stockpot: Necessary for preparing large batches of soups, stews, and stocks.

2. **Baking Sheets and Pans**
   - Baking Sheet: For roasting vegetables, baking chicken, and making sheet pan meals.
   - Casserole Dish: Essential for baking casseroles and other oven dishes.
   - Loaf Pan: For baking whole grain breads and meatloaf.

3. **Steamer Basket**
   - A simple and effective tool for steaming vegetables, preserving their nutrients and flavor.

4. **Colander**
   - For draining pasta, rinsing grains, and washing vegetables and fruits.

Small Appliances

1. **Blender**
   - High-Powered Blender: Useful for making smoothies, soups, and purees. It can also be used for preparing sauces and dressings.

2. **Food Processor**
   - For chopping, slicing, shredding, and mixing. It's a time-saver for tasks like making nut butters, hummus, and finely chopped vegetables.

3. **Slow Cooker or Instant Pot**
   - Slow Cooker: Great for making soups, stews, and slow-cooked meals.

- Instant Pot: Combines multiple functions including pressure cooking, slow cooking, and steaming, making meal prep faster and more convenient.

4. Rice **Cooker or Multi-Cooker**
- Ensures perfectly cooked whole grains like brown rice, quinoa, and farro with minimal effort.

5. Immersion Blender
- Perfect for blending soups and sauces directly in the pot, reducing the need for multiple dishes.

Storage and Organization

1. **Storage Containers**
- Glass or BPA-Free Plastic Containers: For storing leftovers and meal prepping. Various sizes are useful for portion control and organized storage.
- Mason Jars: Great for salads, overnight oats, and storing homemade dressings and sauces.

2. **Herb Keeper**
- Keeps fresh herbs like cilantro, parsley, and basil fresh for longer periods.

3. **Spice Rack**
- Keeps spices organized and easily accessible, encouraging the use of a variety of herbs and spices to enhance flavor without added sodium.

Specialty Tools

1. **Salad Spinner**
   - Efficiently dries leafy greens and herbs, ensuring they stay crisp and fresh.

2. **Mandoline Slicer**
   - For quickly and uniformly slicing vegetables, which is perfect for salads, stir-fries, and garnishes.

3. **Microplane or Zester**
   - Useful for grating citrus zest, garlic, ginger, and hard cheeses to add fresh, vibrant flavors to your dishes.

4. **Digital Food Scale**
   - Helps with accurate portion control and baking, ensuring consistency in your recipes.

Healthy Cooking Accessories

1. **Oil Mister or Spray Bottle**
   - For lightly coating pans and vegetables with oil, reducing overall fat intake while cooking.

2. **Silicone Baking Mats**
   - A non-stick alternative to parchment paper, ideal for baking and roasting with minimal oil.

3. **Oven Thermometer**
   - Ensures your oven is at the correct temperature, which is crucial for consistent cooking and baking results.

Equipping your kitchen with these essential tools and gadgets can make following the DASH diet more convenient and enjoyable. Having the right equipment not only streamlines meal preparation but also encourages healthier cooking practices and portion control. Investing in quality tools can significantly impact your ability to create delicious, nutritious meals that align with the DASH diet principles, ultimately supporting your journey towards better health and well-being.

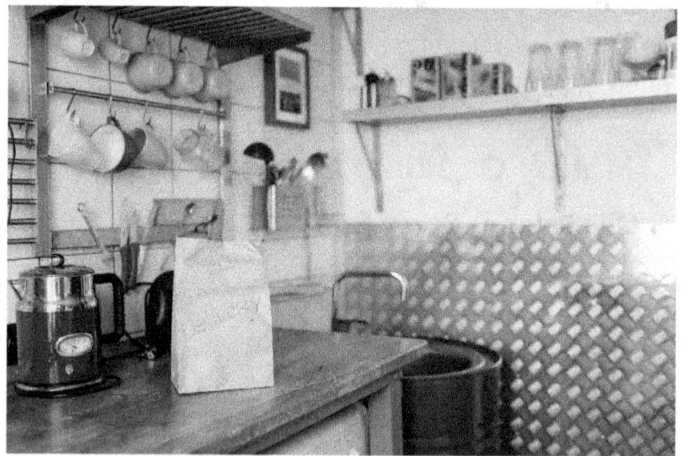

CHAPTER SIX

Stocking Your Pantry: DASH-Friendly Ingredients

A well-stocked pantry is essential for anyone following the DASH (Dietary Approaches to Stop Hypertension) diet. It ensures you have the necessary ingredients on hand to prepare nutritious meals that adhere to the DASH principles.

Friendly ingredients.

1. Whole Grains

Whole grains are a cornerstone of the DASH diet, providing essential fiber, vitamins, and minerals. These complex carbohydrates help maintain stable blood sugar levels and promote heart health.

- Brown Rice: A versatile grain that can be used in salads, stir-fries, and side dishes.
- Quinoa: High in protein and fiber, perfect for salads and as a rice substitute.
- Whole Wheat Pasta: An alternative to refined pasta that adds more nutrients and fiber to your meals.
- Oats: Ideal for breakfast as oatmeal or in baking recipes.
- Barley: Great for soups, stews, and salads.
- Farro: A nutty-tasting grain that works well in salads and side dishes.

- Whole Grain Bread and Tortillas: Look for options with whole grains listed as the first ingredient.

2. Fruits and Vegetables

Fruits and vegetables are rich in vitamins, minerals, antioxidants, and fiber, all of which are crucial for maintaining good health and preventing chronic diseases.

- Canned Vegetables: Choose no-salt-added or low-sodium options.
- Canned Tomatoes: Used in soups, stews, sauces, and casseroles. Opt for no-salt-added varieties.
- Dried Fruits: Look for unsweetened varieties to add to cereals, salads, or as snacks.
- Canned Fruits: Select fruits packed in water or their own juice, avoiding those in syrup.
- Vegetable Juice: Low-sodium vegetable juice can be a quick and easy way to add servings of vegetables to your diet.

3. Legumes and Beans

Legumes and beans are excellent sources of protein, fiber, and essential nutrients. They are adaptable and work well in many different recipes.

- Canned Beans: Black beans, kidney beans, chickpeas, and lentils are great for salads, soups, and stews. Opt for low-sodium or rinse regular canned beans to reduce sodium content.
- Dried Beans and Lentils: Economical and can be cooked in large batches for multiple meals.

4. Lean Proteins

Lean proteins are crucial for muscle maintenance and repair, and they play a key role in a balanced diet.

- Canned Fish: Tuna, salmon, and sardines packed in water provide omega-3 fatty acids and are convenient for quick meals.
- Nut Butters: Peanut butter, almond butter, and other nut butters should be unsweetened and free from hydrogenated oils.
- Canned Chicken: A convenient source of lean protein, useful for salads and quick meals.

5. Healthy Fats

Healthy fats, particularly those from plant sources, are important for heart health. They provide essential fatty acids and help with the absorption of fat-soluble vitamins.

- Olive Oil: Use for cooking, salad dressings, and marinades.
- Canola Oil: Another heart-healthy oil suitable for cooking and baking.
- Nuts and Seeds: Almonds, walnuts, chia seeds, flaxseeds, and sunflower seeds are great for snacks, salads, and adding to baked goods.

6. Dairy and Alternatives

Low-fat and fat-free dairy products provide calcium, vitamin D, and protein without the added saturated fat of full-fat versions.
- Shelf-Stable Milk: Low-fat or fat-free options, as well as plant-based milks like almond, soy, or oat milk.
- Powdered Milk: Can be reconstituted for recipes or used as a protein and calcium booster.

7. Spices and Seasonings

Herbs and spices are essential for adding flavor to your meals without the need for added salt, aligning with the DASH diet's focus on low sodium intake.
- Herbs and Spices: Basil, oregano, thyme, rosemary, cumin, coriander, paprika, turmeric, cinnamon, and nutmeg.
- Salt-Free Seasoning Blends: Pre-mixed blends like Mrs. Dash or other no-salt-added options can enhance the flavor of your dishes.
- Vinegars: Balsamic, apple cider, red wine, and rice vinegar are versatile and can be used in dressings, marinades, and sauces.

8. **Condiments and Sauces**

Choose condiments and sauces wisely to avoid hidden sodium and added sugars.
- Mustard: Yellow, Dijon, or whole grain mustard adds flavor with minimal calories.
- Hot Sauce: Opt for low-sodium varieties.
- Soy Sauce: Use low-sodium versions to control salt intake.
- Tomato Sauce: Choose no-salt-added or make your own to control sodium levels.
- Salsa: Look for low-sodium options or make fresh salsa at home.

9. **Baking Supplies**

Having the right baking supplies on hand can help you prepare healthier baked goods.
- Whole Wheat Flour: Use in place of or in combination with white flour for added fiber and nutrients.
- Baking Powder and Baking Soda: Essential for leavening.
- Honey and Maple Syrup: Natural sweeteners to use in moderation.
- Unsweetened Applesauce: A healthy substitute for oil or butter in baking.

10. **Snacks**

Snacking healthily might help you avoid overindulging during meals and maintain a steady energy level.

- Popcorn: Air-popped and without added butter or salt.
- Whole Grain Crackers: Choose options with minimal ingredients and no added sugar.
- Dried Fruit and Nut Mixes: Make your own mixes to control the ingredients and portion sizes.

Stocking your pantry with these DASH-friendly ingredients ensures you have the foundation to prepare healthy, delicious meals that support your dietary goals. By keeping these staples on hand, you can easily adhere to the principles of the DASH diet, promoting better heart health and overall well-being. Investing time in organizing and maintaining a well-stocked pantry can significantly simplify meal preparation and make healthy eating more accessible and sustainable.

Reading Food Labels: What to Look For

Reading food labels is a crucial skill for anyone following the DASH (Dietary Approaches to Stop Hypertension) diet. Understanding the information on food packaging can help you make informed choices that align with the DASH principles of reducing sodium, saturated fats, and added sugars, while increasing nutrients like potassium, calcium, and fiber.

1. **Serving Size and Servings Per Container**

The first place to start when reading a food label is the serving size and the number of servings per container.

- Serving Size: This is the amount of food that is considered one serving. It's essential to compare the serving size to how much you actually eat. If you consume double the serving size, you need to double all the nutritional values listed.
- Servings Per Container: This indicates the total number of servings in the product. Understanding this helps in accurately calculating the total intake of nutrients.

2. **Calories**

An indicator of how much energy a portion of this dish contains is its calorie count.

- Total Calories: Check the calories per serving, especially if you are monitoring your caloric intake to manage your weight.
- Calories from Fat: While not always listed, it can give insight into how much of the calorie content comes from fat.

3. **Nutrients to Limit**

Certain nutrients should be limited in the DASH diet due to their potential negative impact on heart health.

- Total Fat: Look at the amount of total fat and pay particular attention to the types of fat.
  - Saturated Fat: Aim to keep your intake low. High levels of saturated fat can increase blood cholesterol and the risk of heart disease.
  - Trans Fat: Avoid trans fats as much as possible. They may lower HDL and raise LDL, the harmful kind of cholesterol.
- Cholesterol: Excessive intake of cholesterol can contribute to heart disease. Aim for less than 300 mg per day.
- Sodium: Key for the DASH diet, which emphasizes reducing sodium intake. Look for foods with low sodium content. Aim for less than 2,300 mg per day, ideally reducing to 1,500 mg for greater heart health benefits.

4. **Nutrients to Get More Of**

The DASH diet encourages higher intake of certain nutrients to promote overall health and manage blood pressure.

- Dietary Fiber: High fiber intake is associated with better digestion and lower cholesterol levels. Aim for 25-30 grams per day. Foods with 5 grams or more per serving are considered high in fiber.
- Vitamin D: Important for bone health and immune function.

- Calcium: Essential for bone health. Aim for
1,000-1,300 mg per day.
- Iron: Necessary for carrying oxygen in the blood.
Aim to get sufficient iron, particularly for women
who may need more.
- Potassium: Helps to balance sodium levels and
maintain healthy blood pressure. Aim for 4,700 mg
per day.

5. Total Carbohydrates

Carbohydrates are a primary energy source. The
total carbohydrate section includes fiber and
sugars.
- Dietary Fiber: As mentioned, aim for foods high in
fiber.
- Total Sugars: Check both the natural and added
sugars.
  - Added Sugars: Limit added sugars to less than
10% of your daily calories. High added sugars can
contribute to weight gain and increased risk of
chronic diseases.

6. Protein

Protein is essential for building and repairing
tissues. The DASH diet encourages lean sources of
protein, such as fish, poultry, legumes, and nuts.
Aim for a balance of protein from both animal and
plant sources.

7. **Vitamins and Minerals**

Check the Percent Daily Value (%DV) to understand how much a serving contributes to your daily intake of vitamins and minerals.
- Vitamins A and C, Calcium, and Iron: These are often listed, but pay attention to any other vitamins and minerals that may be highlighted. Aim for foods that provide a higher %DV of these nutrients.

8. **Ingredient List**

A peek at the ingredient list tells you exactly what's in your dish. The ingredients are arranged by weight in descending order.
- First Three Ingredients: These make up the majority of the product. Look for whole foods like whole grains, vegetables, fruits, and lean proteins.
- Avoid Added Sugars and Refined Grains: Ingredients like high fructose corn syrup, cane sugar, and white flour are less desirable.
- Watch for Additives: Be mindful of preservatives, artificial colors, and flavors. Choose foods with minimal processing and fewer additives.

9. **Claims on Packaging**

Food packaging often includes claims that can be misleading. Here's how to interpret them:
- "Low Sodium": Denotes a serving size of 140 mg or less of sodium.
- "Reduced Sodium": Contains at least 25% less sodium than the regular product.

- "No Salt Added": No salt is added during processing, but it does not mean the product is sodium-free.
- "Whole Grain": Look for "100% whole grain" or check the ingredient list to ensure whole grains are the primary ingredient.
- "Organic": Refers to the farming practices used. Organic foods may have fewer pesticides and additives but can still contain sugars and fats.
- "Natural": This term is not well-regulated and does not necessarily mean healthy. Always read the ingredient list.

10. Special Considerations

For those with specific dietary needs or preferences, here are additional tips:
- Allergens: Look for allergen statements if you have food allergies or intolerances.
- Gluten-Free: For those with celiac disease or gluten sensitivity, ensure products are labeled gluten-free.
- Vegan or Vegetarian: Check for animal-derived ingredients if you follow a plant-based diet.

Reading food labels is a vital skill for maintaining a healthy diet, particularly when following the DASH diet. By understanding serving sizes, calories, and the balance of nutrients, you can make more informed food choices that support your health goals. Always remember to look beyond marketing claims and focus on the actual nutritional content and ingredient list to ensure you're selecting the healthiest options available. With practice, reading food labels will become second nature, helping you to navigate the grocery store with confidence and make choices that benefit your long-term health.

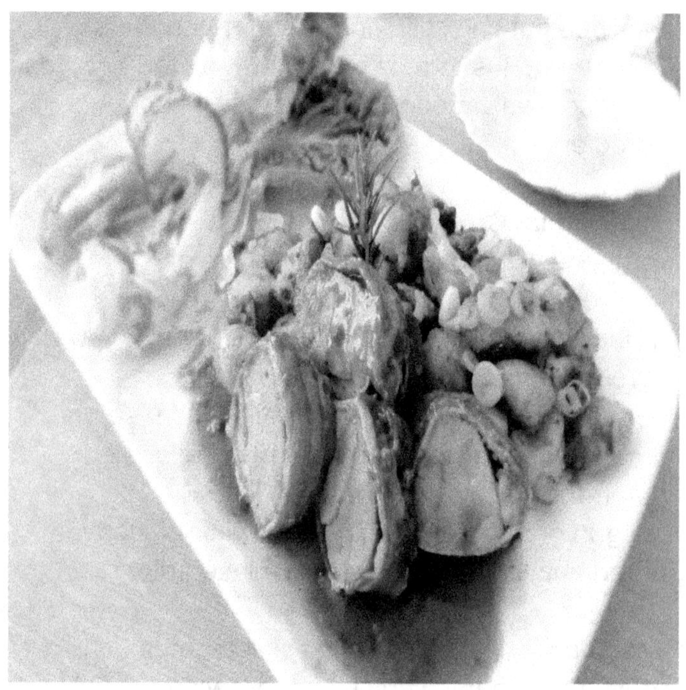

CHAPTER SEVEN

BREAKFAST RECIPES

Energizing Smoothies and Juices for Breakfast

Starting your day with a nutritious and energizing breakfast is essential, especially when following the DASH (Dietary Approaches to Stop Hypertension) diet. Smoothies and juices can be convenient options packed with vitamins, minerals, and fiber to kickstart your morning. Here's are some energizing smoothies and juices that align with DASH diet principles:

Benefits of Smoothies and Juices
1.Nutrient-Rich: Packed with vitamins, minerals, and antioxidants from fruits, vegetables, and other ingredients.

2. Hydration: Helps to start your day hydrated, especially if made with water or coconut water.

3. Convenience: Quick and easy to prepare, making them ideal for busy mornings.

4. Digestion: Smoothies and juices can aid digestion and promote gut health, especially if they include fiber-rich ingredients.

Tips for Making Energizing Smoothies and Juices

1. Balance Your Ingredients: Include a mix of fruits, vegetables, protein, and healthy fats for a well-rounded breakfast.

2. Watch Sugar Content: Limit added sugars by using whole fruits and vegetables as sweeteners.

3. Add Protein: Incorporate sources like Greek yogurt, nut butter, or protein powder to help keep you full until your next meal.

4. Include Fiber: Fiber-rich ingredients like chia seeds, flaxseeds, or leafy greens help with digestion and satiety.

Energizing Smoothie Recipes

1. **Green Power Smoothie**
- Ingredients:
  - A cup of spinach or kale leaves
  - Half a frozen banana, for a creamier consistency
  - 1/2 cup frozen pineapple chunks
  - 1/2 cup Greek yogurt
  - 1 tablespoon chia seeds
  - One cup of unsweetened coconut water or almond milk

- Instructions:
    1. Fill a blender with all the ingredients.
    2. Blend until smooth and creamy.
    3. Transfer to a glass and start sipping right away.

2. Berry Blast Smoothie
- Ingredients:
  - 1/2 cup of mixed berries, including raspberries, blueberries, and strawberries
  - 1/2 cup plain Greek yogurt
  - One tablespoon of maple syrup or honey (optional, depending on desired sweetness)
  - 1 tablespoon ground flaxseeds
  - 1/2 cup of unsweetened coconut water or almond milk

- Instructions:
    1. Fill a blender with all the ingredients.
    2. Blend until smooth.
    3. Taste and adjust sweetness if necessary.
    4. Transfer into a glass for serving.

Energizing Juice Recipes

1. Citrus Ginger Juice
- Ingredients:
  - 2 oranges, peeled and segmented
  - 1 lemon, peeled and segmented
  - A 1-inch piece of raw, peeled ginger
  - 1 cup water or coconut water (optional, for desired consistency)

- Instructions:
   1. Place all ingredients in a juicer or blender.
   2. Blend or juice until smooth.
   3. Strain the mixture if desired for a smoother texture.
   4. Serve chilled over ice.

2. **Green Detox Juice**
- Ingredients:
   - 1 cucumber, peeled and chopped
   - 2 cups spinach leaves
   - One cored and cut green apple
   - 1/2 lemon, peeled
   - A 1-inch piece of raw, peeled ginger

- Instructions:
   1. Use a juicer to juice every item.
   2. Stir well and serve immediately over ice.

 Additional Tips
- Prep Ahead: Pre-cut fruits and vegetables and store them in the freezer for quick and easy smoothie preparation.

- Variety: Experiment with different combinations of fruits, vegetables, and herbs to keep your breakfasts exciting and varied.

- Portion Control: Pay attention to portion sizes and avoid oversized servings, especially with calorie-dense ingredients like nut butters or sweeteners.

Energizing smoothies and juices are excellent options for a nutritious breakfast that supports the DASH diet principles. They provide a quick and convenient way to incorporate a variety of fruits, vegetables, and other wholesome ingredients into your morning routine. By following these recipes and tips, you can start your day with a refreshing and nutrient-packed beverage that fuels your body and helps you maintain optimal health and energy throughout the day.

Wholesome Oatmeal and Porridge Breakfast Recipes

Oatmeal and porridge are classic breakfast options that are not only delicious but also nutritious, making them perfect for those following the DASH (Dietary Approaches to Stop Hypertension) diet. Packed with fiber, vitamins, and minerals, these recipes provide sustained energy and support heart health.

Benefits of Oatmeal and Porridge

1. High in Fiber: Supports digestive health and helps keep you full longer.

2. Rich in Nutrients: Provides essential vitamins and minerals like iron, magnesium, and B vitamins.

3. Heart-Healthy: Oats contain beta-glucan, a type of soluble fiber linked to improved heart health and cholesterol levels.

Tips for Making Wholesome Oatmeal and Porridge

1. Choose Whole Grains: Opt for rolled oats, steel-cut oats, or whole grain porridge mixes for maximum nutritional benefits.

2. Control Sweeteners: Use natural sweeteners like honey, maple syrup, or fresh fruits instead of refined sugars.

3. Add Protein: Incorporate sources like nuts, seeds, Greek yogurt, or milk to increase protein content and enhance satiety.

4. Boost Flavor: Experiment with spices like cinnamon, nutmeg, or vanilla extract for added flavor without extra calories.

Wholesome Oatmeal Recipes

1. **Classic Rolled Oats**
- Ingredients:
  - 1/2 cup rolled oats
  - A cup of water, plant-based milk, or dairy
  - Pinch of salt
  - Optional toppings: Fresh berries, sliced banana, nuts (almonds, walnuts), seeds (chia seeds, flaxseeds), honey or maple syrup

- Instructions:
  1. In a small saucepan, bring water or milk to a boil.
  2. Stir in rolled oats and salt.
  3. Reduce heat to low and simmer for 5-7 minutes, stirring occasionally, until oats are creamy and tender.
  4. Remove from heat and let stand for a minute to thicken.
  5. Serve hot, topped with your favorite toppings.

2. Overnight Oats
- Ingredients:
  - 1/2 cup rolled oats
  - 1/2 cup Greek yogurt
  - 1/2 cup milk (dairy or plant-based)
  - 1 tablespoon chia seeds (optional)
  - 1/2 teaspoon vanilla extract
  - Optional sweeteners: Honey, maple syrup, or mashed banana
  - Optional toppings: Fresh fruits, nuts, seeds

- Instructions:
  1. In a jar or container, combine rolled oats, Greek yogurt, milk, chia seeds (if using), vanilla extract, and sweeteners.
  2. Stir well until all ingredients are thoroughly mixed.
  3. For at least four hours, preferably overnight, cover and refrigerate.

4. In the morning, stir and adjust consistency with additional milk if desired.

5. Top with fruits, nuts, and seeds before serving.

Wholesome Porridge Recipes

1. **Quinoa Porridge**

- Ingredients:
  - 1/2 cup quinoa, rinsed
  - A cup of water, plant-based milk, or dairy
  - Pinch of salt
  - Optional sweeteners: Honey, maple syrup
  - Optional toppings: Fresh fruits, nuts (almonds, walnuts), seeds (pumpkin seeds, sunflower seeds), cinnamon

- Instructions:
  1. In a small saucepan, bring water or milk to a boil.
  2. Add quinoa and salt, reduce heat to low, and simmer covered for 15-20 minutes, or until quinoa is tender and liquid is absorbed.
  3. Remove from heat and let stand for a few minutes to thicken.
  4. Stir in sweeteners if desired.
  5. Serve warm, topped with fruits, nuts, seeds, and a sprinkle of cinnamon.

2. **Millet Porridge**

- Ingredients:
  - 1/2 cup millet
  - Two cups of water, plant-based milk, or dairy
  - Pinch of salt
  - Optional sweeteners: Honey, maple syrup
  - Optional toppings: Fresh berries, sliced banana, nuts (pecans, almonds), coconut flakes

- Instructions:
  1. Rinse millet under cold water.
  2. In a saucepan, bring water or milk to a boil.
  3. Add millet and salt, reduce heat to low, and simmer covered for 20-25 minutes, stirring occasionally, until millet is tender and liquid is absorbed.
  4. Remove from heat and let stand for a few minutes to thicken.
  5. Stir in sweeteners if desired.
  6. Serve warm, topped with fruits, nuts, and coconut flakes.

Additional Tips

- Batch Cooking: Prepare larger quantities of oatmeal or porridge and store leftovers in the refrigerator for quick breakfasts throughout the week.

- Customization: Experiment with different grains, liquids, and toppings to keep your breakfasts interesting and varied.

- Nutrient Boost: Add ground flaxseeds, hemp seeds, or spirulina powder for an extra nutrient boost.

Wholesome oatmeal and porridge recipes are versatile, nutritious, and satisfying breakfast options that align perfectly with the DASH diet principles. By incorporating whole grains, healthy proteins, and a variety of toppings, you can create delicious breakfasts that support heart health, provide sustained energy, and keep you full until your next meal. Whether you prefer classic oats or adventurous porridge options, these recipes are sure to become staples in your morning routine, helping you start your day on a healthy and delicious note.

Healthy Breakfast Bowls

Breakfast bowls are a versatile and nutritious way to start your day, especially when following the DASH (Dietary Approaches to Stop Hypertension) diet. These bowls typically combine a variety of wholesome ingredients like whole grains, fruits, vegetables, nuts, seeds, and lean proteins to create a balanced meal that supports heart health and provides sustained energy.

Benefits of Breakfast Bowls
1. Nutrient-Dense: Packed with essential vitamins, minerals, and antioxidants from a variety of ingredients.

2. Customizable: Easily tailored to personal preferences and dietary needs.

3. Balanced: Provides a mix of carbohydrates, protein, and healthy fats to keep you full and satisfied.

Tips for Making Healthy Breakfast Bowls
1. Choose Whole Grains: Opt for whole grains like quinoa, brown rice, oats, or barley as the base for added fiber and nutrients.

2. Incorporate Protein: Include lean protein sources such as Greek yogurt, eggs, tofu, or beans to promote satiety and muscle health.

3. Add Colorful Vegetables and Fruits: Pack your bowl with a variety of colorful vegetables and fruits for vitamins, minerals, and antioxidants.

4. Healthy Fats: Include sources like nuts, seeds, avocado, or olive oil to provide essential fatty acids and enhance flavor.

Healthy Breakfast Bowl Recipes

1. **Mediterranean Quinoa Breakfast Bowl**
- Ingredients:
  - 1/2 cup cooked quinoa
  - 1/4 cup cherry tomatoes, halved
  - 1/4 cup cucumber, diced
  - 2 tablespoons Kalamata olives, sliced
  - 1/4 cup chickpeas, rinsed and drained
  - 1/4 avocado, sliced
  - 1 tablespoon feta cheese, crumbled
  - Fresh parsley, chopped (for garnish)
  - Lemon wedge (optional, for drizzling)

- Instructions:
  1. In a bowl, layer cooked quinoa as the base.
  2. Arrange cherry tomatoes, cucumber, olives, chickpeas, and avocado on top.
  3. Sprinkle with feta cheese and fresh parsley.
  4. Drizzle with olive oil and a squeeze of lemon juice if desired.
  5. Serve immediately and enjoy!

2. **Berry and Yogurt Breakfast Bowl**
- Ingredients:
  - 1/2 cup plain Greek yogurt
  - 1/2 cup of mixed berries, including raspberries, blueberries, and strawberries
  - 1/4 cup granola (choose low-sugar or homemade)
  - One tablespoon of ground flaxseeds or chia seeds

- One tablespoon (optional, for sweetness) of
honey or maple syrup
  - Fresh mint leaves (for garnish)

- Instructions:
  1. Spoon Greek yogurt into a bowl as the base.
  2. Add granola and mixed berries on top.
  3. Sprinkle with chia seeds or ground flaxseeds.
  4. Drizzle with honey or maple syrup if desired.
  5. Garnish with fresh mint leaves.
  6. Serve immediately and enjoy!

Additional Healthy Breakfast Bowl Ideas

1. **Egg and Vegetable Breakfast Bowl**
- Ingredients:
  - 1/2 cup of brown rice or cooked quinoa
  - 1 egg, poached or fried
  - 1 cup spinach or kale, sautéed
  - 1/4 cup cherry tomatoes, halved
  - 1/4 avocado, sliced
  - Sriracha or hot sauce (optional, for added spice)
  - Salt and pepper to taste

- Instructions:
  1. Layer cooked quinoa or brown rice as the base
of the bowl.
  2. Top with sautéed spinach or kale, cherry
tomatoes, and sliced avocado.
  3. Place the poached or fried egg on top.
  4. Season with salt, pepper, and drizzle with
sriracha or hot sauce if desired.

5. Serve immediately and enjoy!

2. **Tropical Smoothie Bowl**
- Ingredients:
  - 1 frozen banana
  - 1/2 cup frozen mango chunks
  - 1/2 cup frozen pineapple chunks
  - 1/2 cup plain Greek yogurt
  - 1/4 cup unsweetened almond milk or coconut water
  - Toppings: Fresh kiwi slices, shredded coconut, chia seeds, granola

- Instructions:
  1. In a blender, combine frozen banana, mango chunks, pineapple chunks, Greek yogurt, and almond milk or coconut water.
  2. Blend until smooth and creamy, adding more liquid if needed.
  3. Pour into a bowl and top with kiwi slices, shredded coconut, chia seeds, and granola.
  4. Serve immediately with a spoon and enjoy!

Quick and Easy Breakfast Ideas

Mornings can be hectic, but starting your day with a nutritious breakfast is essential for energy and focus. These quick and easy breakfast ideas are perfect for those busy mornings, designed to be prepared in minutes without compromising on flavor or nutrition.

Benefits of Quick and Easy Breakfasts
1. Time-Saving: Ready in minutes, perfect for busy schedules.

2. Nutritious: Provide essential nutrients to fuel your day.

3. Versatile: Easily customizable to suit personal preferences and dietary needs.

Quick and Easy Breakfast Ideas

1. **Avocado Toast**
- Ingredients:
  - 1-2 slices whole grain bread, toasted
  - 1 ripe avocado
  - Salt and pepper to taste

- Optional toppings: Sliced tomatoes,
microgreens, poached egg, feta cheese

- Instructions:
  1. Until golden brown, toast the whole grain bread.
  2. Mash the ripe avocado and spread it evenly on
the toasted bread.
  3. Sprinkle it with salt and pepper.
  4. Add optional toppings such as sliced tomatoes,
microgreens, poached egg, or crumbled feta
cheese.
  5. Serve immediately and enjoy!

2. Yogurt Parfait

- Ingredients:
  - Half a cup of plain or flavored Greek yogurt
  - 1/4 cup granola (choose low-sugar or
homemade)
  - 1/2 cup of mixed berries, including raspberries,
blueberries, and strawberries
  - Optional toppings: Honey or maple syrup, nuts
(almonds, walnuts), chia seeds

- Instructions:
  1. Arrange mixed berries, Greek yogurt, and
granola in a bowl or glass.
  2. Repeat layers until ingredients are used up.
  3. If preferred, drizzle with maple syrup or honey.
  4. Sprinkle with nuts and chia seeds for added
crunch and nutrients.
  5. Serve immediately with a spoon and enjoy!

3. **Fruit and Nut Butter Wrap**
- Ingredients:
  - 1 whole wheat or whole grain wrap
  - 2 tablespoons nut butter (peanut butter, almond butter)
  - 1 banana, sliced
  - Optional additions: Honey or maple syrup, cinnamon

- Instructions:
  1. Spread nut butter evenly over the wrap.
  2. Place sliced bananas on one side of the wrap.
  3. Drizzle with honey or maple syrup and sprinkle with cinnamon if desired.
  4. Roll up the wrap tightly, cut in half if desired, and serve immediately.

4. **Overnight Chia Seed Pudding**
- Ingredients:
  - 1/4 cup chia seeds
  - A cup of almond or coconut milk without sugar added.
  - 1/2 teaspoon vanilla extract
  - Optional sweeteners: Honey, maple syrup, or mashed banana
  - Optional toppings include shredded coconut, sliced almonds, and fresh berries.

- Instructions:
  1. In a jar or container, combine chia seeds, almond milk, and vanilla extract.
  2. Stir well until chia seeds are evenly distributed.

3. Cover and refrigerate overnight or for at least 4 hours until thickened.

4. Stir again before serving and adjust consistency with additional milk if desired.

5. Top with fresh berries, sliced almonds, and shredded coconut before serving.

5. **Smoothie**

- Ingredients:
  - A cup of spinach or kale leaves
  - Half a frozen banana, for a creamier consistency
  - 1/2 cup of frozen blueberries, raspberries, and strawberries
  - Half a cup of plain or flavored Greek yogurt
  - One tablespoon of ground flaxseeds or chia seeds
  - One cup of unsweetened coconut water or almond milk

- Instructions:
  1. Fill a blender with all the ingredients.
  2. Blend until smooth and creamy.
  3. Transfer to a glass and start sipping right away.

Additional Tips

- Meal Prep: Prepare ingredients in advance, such as chopping fruits or portioning out ingredients, to save time in the morning.

- Customization: Experiment with different combinations of fruits, vegetables, and proteins to keep breakfasts interesting and varied.

- Portion Control: Pay attention to portion sizes and avoid oversized servings, especially with calorie-dense ingredients like nut butters or sweeteners.

Quick and easy breakfast ideas provide a convenient way to fuel your body with essential nutrients without sacrificing taste or health benefits. Whether you prefer savory or sweet options, these recipes are designed to fit into busy lifestyles while promoting overall well-being. By incorporating these ideas into your morning routine, you can start each day feeling energized, satisfied, and ready to tackle whatever lies ahead.

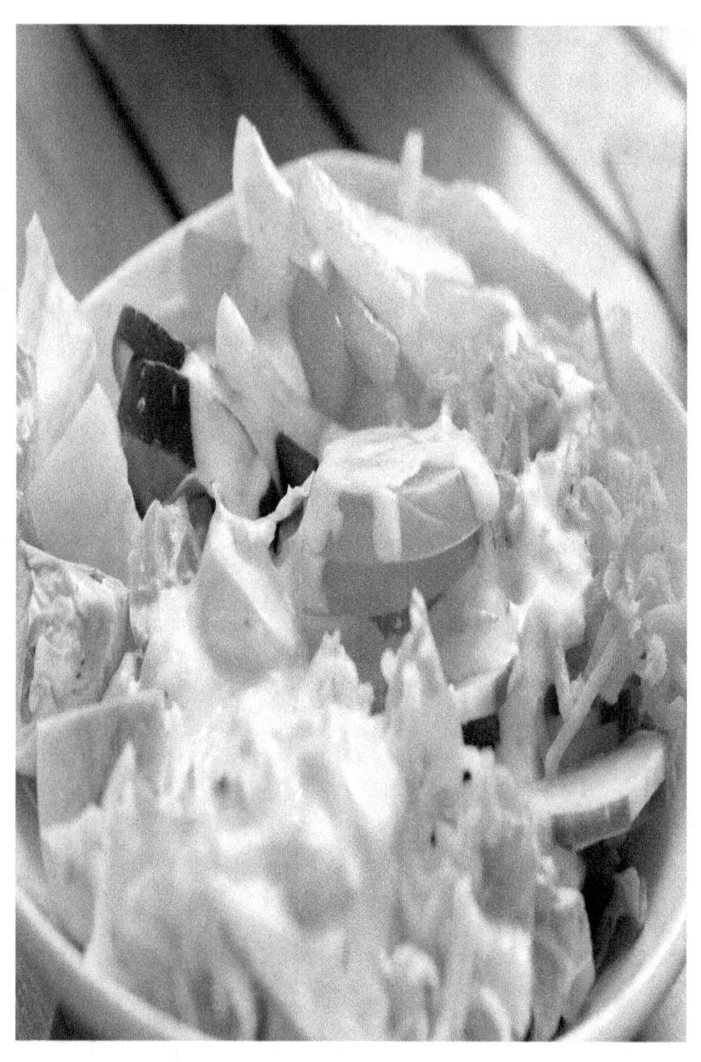

CHAPTER EIGHT

Lunch recipes

Fresh and Flavorful Salad Lunch Recipes

Salads are not only refreshing and satisfying but also a great way to incorporate a variety of fresh ingredients into your diet. These lunch salad recipes are packed with nutrients, flavors, and textures, making them perfect for a wholesome meal that aligns with the principles of the DASH (Dietary Approaches to Stop Hypertension) diet.

Benefits of Fresh and Flavorful Salads

1. Nutrient-Rich: Loaded with vitamins, minerals, and antioxidants from fresh vegetables, fruits, and other wholesome ingredients.

2. Hydration: Many salad ingredients have high water content, contributing to hydration.

3. Versatility: Easily customizable with a wide range of vegetables, fruits, proteins, and dressings.

Tips for Making Fresh and Flavorful Salads

1. Choose Leafy Greens: Start with a base of nutrient-dense leafy greens such as spinach, kale, arugula, or mixed greens.

2. Add Colorful Vegetables and Fruits: Incorporate a variety of colorful vegetables like tomatoes, bell peppers, cucumbers, carrots, and fruits like berries or citrus for added flavor and nutrients.

3. Include Protein: Boost satiety and muscle health by adding lean proteins such as grilled chicken, tofu, chickpeas, beans, quinoa, or nuts.

4. Healthy Fats: Enhance flavor and provide essential fatty acids with sources like avocado, olive oil, nuts, or seeds.

Fresh and Flavorful Salad Recipes

1. **Mediterranean Quinoa Salad**
- Ingredients:
  - 1 cup cooked quinoa, cooled
  - 1 cup cherry tomatoes, halved
  - 1 cucumber, diced
  - 1/4 cup finely diced red onion
  - 1/4 cup Kalamata olives, sliced
  - 1/4 cup feta cheese, crumbled
  - Fresh parsley, chopped

- Instructions:
   1. In a large bowl, combine cooked quinoa, cherry tomatoes, cucumber, red onion, olives, and feta cheese.

   2. Add a lemon juice and olive oil drizzle.

   3. For seasoning add salt and pepper to taste.

   4. Toss gently to combine.

   5. Before serving, garnish with fresh parsley.

2. **Grilled Chicken and Avocado Salad**
- Ingredients:
   - 2 cups mixed greens (spinach, arugula, or mixed greens)
   - 1 grilled chicken breast, sliced
   - 1/2 avocado, sliced
   - 1/2 cup cherry tomatoes, halved
   - 1/4 cup cucumber, sliced
   - 1/4 cup chopped red bell pepper
   - 2 tablespoons sunflower seeds or sliced almonds

- Instructions:
   1. Arrange mixed greens on a serving plate.
   2. Top with grilled chicken, avocado, cherry tomatoes, cucumber, and red bell pepper.
   3. Sprinkle with sunflower seeds or sliced almonds.

4. Drizzle with balsamic vinaigrette or your favorite dressing.

5. Serve immediately and enjoy!

3. **Citrus and Quinoa Salad**
- Ingredients:
  - 1 cup cooked quinoa, cooled
  - 1 orange, peeled and segmented
  - 1/2 grapefruit, peeled and segmented
  - 1/4 cup pomegranate seeds
  - 1/4 cup of fresh mint leaves, cut finely
  - 1/4 cup feta cheese, crumbled
  - Mixed greens (optional)

- Instructions:
  1. Put cooked quinoa, feta cheese, orange and grapefruit segments, pomegranate seeds, and mint leaves in a big bowl.
  2. If desired, serve over a bed of mixed greens.
  3. Drizzle with a citrus vinaigrette or olive oil and lemon juice.
  4. Toss gently to combine.
  5. Serve immediately and enjoy!

Additional Tips
- Prep Ahead: Prepare ingredients in advance and store them separately to assemble salads quickly during busy weekdays.

- Dressing on the Side: Serve dressings on the side to control portions and prevent salads from becoming soggy if not consumed immediately.

- Experiment with Ingredients: Customize salads with seasonal vegetables, fruits, herbs, and proteins to keep meals exciting and varied.

Fresh and flavorful salads are excellent options for a nutritious and satisfying lunch that supports the DASH diet principles. By incorporating a variety of vegetables, fruits, proteins, and healthy fats into your salads, you can create delicious and wholesome meals that promote overall health and well-being. Whether you prefer Mediterranean-inspired flavors or vibrant citrus combinations, these salad recipes are sure to elevate your lunchtime routine with nutrient-rich ingredients and delightful flavors.

Satisfying Sandwiches and Wraps

Sandwiches and wraps are convenient and satisfying lunch options that can be easily customized to fit the DASH (Dietary Approaches to Stop Hypertension) diet principles. These recipes focus on using wholesome ingredients like lean proteins, whole grains, and plenty of vegetables to create delicious and nutritious meals.

Benefits of Satisfying Sandwiches and Wraps
1. Balanced Nutrition: Provide a mix of carbohydrates, proteins, and healthy fats.

2. Customizable: Easily adjust ingredients to suit personal taste preferences and dietary needs.

3. Portable: Ideal for on-the-go lunches or meal prepping.

Tips for Making Satisfying Sandwiches and Wraps

1. Choose Whole Grain Bread or Wraps: Opt for whole grain options to increase fiber content and promote satiety.

2. Incorporate Lean Proteins: Use lean meats (turkey, chicken), seafood, tofu, or legumes (beans, chickpeas) for protein.

3. Load Up on Vegetables: Add plenty of fresh vegetables like lettuce, spinach, tomatoes, cucumbers, bell peppers, and avocado for added nutrients and crunch.

4. Use Healthy Spreads: Choose spreads like hummus, guacamole, or Greek yogurt-based sauces instead of high-fat condiments.

Satisfying Sandwich and Wrap Recipes

1. **Turkey Avocado Wrap**
- Ingredients:
  - Whole wheat or spinach wrap
  - 3 ounces sliced turkey breast
  - 1/4 avocado, mashed

- Handful of spinach leaves
- Sliced tomatoes
- Sliced cucumbers
- Mustard or Greek yogurt-based dressing

- Instructions:
  1. Lay the wrap flat and spread mashed avocado evenly over it.
  2. Layer with sliced turkey breast, spinach leaves, tomatoes, and cucumbers.
  3. Drizzle with mustard or Greek yogurt-based dressing.
  4. Roll up tightly, cut in half if desired, and serve immediately.

2. Mediterranean Veggie Sandwich
- Ingredients:
  - Whole grain bread slices
  - Hummus (store-bought or homemade)
  - Sliced cucumber
  - Sliced bell peppers (red or yellow)
  - Sliced tomatoes
  - Red onion slices
  - Fresh spinach or arugula leaves

- Instructions:
  1. Slather a large slice of bread with hummus.
  2. Layer with cucumber slices, bell peppers, tomatoes, red onion slices, and spinach or arugula leaves.
  3. Place another piece of bread on top.

4. Press gently together, cut in half if desired, and serve.

3. **Grilled Chicken Caesar Wrap**
- Ingredients:
  - Whole wheat or spinach wrap
  - Grilled chicken breast, sliced
  - Romaine lettuce leaves
  - Shaved Parmesan cheese
  - Caesar dressing (store-bought or homemade)

- Instructions:
  1. Lay the wrap flat and layer with romaine lettuce leaves.
  2. Arrange sliced grilled chicken breast on top.
  3. Sprinkle with shaved Parmesan cheese.
  4. Drizzle with Caesar dressing.
  5. Roll up tightly, cut in half if desired, and serve immediately.

Additional Tips
- Add Fresh Herbs: Incorporate fresh herbs like basil, cilantro, or mint for added flavor and nutrients.

- Toast or Grill: Toast sandwiches or grill wraps for added texture and warmth.

- Packaging for Portability: Wrap sandwiches and wraps tightly in parchment paper or foil for easy transport.

Satisfying sandwiches and wraps are versatile lunch options that can be tailored to meet your dietary goals while providing essential nutrients and flavors. Whether you prefer a classic turkey avocado wrap, a Mediterranean veggie sandwich, or a grilled chicken Caesar wrap, these recipes offer delicious ways to enjoy a balanced meal on busy weekdays or leisurely weekends. By choosing wholesome ingredients and experimenting with different combinations, you can create satisfying lunches that keep you fueled and satisfied throughout the day

Hearty Soups and Stews for Lunch

Hearty soups and stews are comforting, nutritious, and perfect for a satisfying lunch that aligns with the principles of the DASH (Dietary Approaches to Stop Hypertension) diet. These recipes are packed with wholesome ingredients like vegetables, lean proteins, and whole grains, providing a balanced meal that supports heart health and overall well-being. Here's a comprehensive guide to creating hearty soups and stews:

Benefits of Hearty Soups and Stews
1. Nutrient-Dense: Rich in vitamins, minerals, and antioxidants from a variety of vegetables and ingredients.

2. Filling and Satisfying: Provide warmth and comfort while promoting satiety.

3. Versatile: Can be prepared in advance and easily customized with different ingredients.

Tips for Making Hearty Soups and Stews
1. Start with a Flavorful Base: Use broth, tomatoes, or coconut milk for a flavorful and nutritious base.

2. Include Lean Proteins: Add lean proteins such as chicken breast, turkey, beans, lentils, or tofu to increase protein content.

3. Add Whole Grains: Incorporate whole grains like quinoa, brown rice, barley, or whole wheat pasta for fiber and complex carbohydrates.

4. Pack with Vegetables: Load up on a variety of vegetables like carrots, celery, onions, bell peppers, spinach, and kale for vitamins and minerals.

Hearty Soup and Stew Recipes

1. **Chicken and Vegetable Quinoa Soup**
- Ingredients:
  - 1 tablespoon olive oil
  - 1 onion, chopped
  - 2 garlic cloves, minced
  - 2 carrots, diced
  - 2 celery stalks, diced
  - 1 red bell pepper, diced
  - One cup of chopped tomatoes (fresh or canned)
  - 1 teaspoon dried thyme
  - 1 teaspoon dried rosemary
  - 1/2 teaspoon paprika
  - 6 cups low-sodium chicken broth
  - 1 cup quinoa, rinsed
  - 2 cups cooked chicken breast, shredded
  - Salt and pepper to taste
  - Fresh parsley, chopped (for garnish)

- Instructions:
  1. Heat the olive oil in a big pot over medium heat. Add the garlic and onion and sauté until tender.

  2. Add carrots, celery, and bell pepper. Cook for 5-7 minutes until vegetables begin to soften.

  3. Stir in diced tomatoes, dried thyme, rosemary, and paprika. Cook for another 2 minutes.

4. Add the chicken broth and heat until it boils.

5. Add quinoa and reduce heat to low. Simmer for 15-20 minutes until quinoa is cooked and vegetables are tender.

6. Stir in shredded chicken breast. Season with salt and pepper to taste.

7. Ladle soup into bowls, garnish with chopped parsley, and serve hot.

2. **Lentil and Vegetable Stew**
- Ingredients:
  - 1 tablespoon olive oil
  - 1 onion, chopped
  - 2 garlic cloves, minced
  - 2 carrots, diced
  - 2 celery stalks, diced
  - 1 red bell pepper, diced
  - One cup of rinsed dried green or brown lentils
  - 1 teaspoon ground cumin
  - 1 teaspoon ground coriander
  - 1/2 teaspoon smoked paprika
  - 6 cups vegetable broth
  - One 14-oz can of chopped tomatoes
  - 2 cups spinach leaves
  - Salt and pepper to taste
  - Fresh cilantro, chopped (for garnish)

- Instructions:
  1. Heat the olive oil in a big pot over medium heat. Add the garlic and onion and sauté until tender.

  2. Add carrots, celery, and bell pepper. Cook for 5-7 minutes until vegetables begin to soften.

  3. Stir in lentils, ground cumin, coriander, and smoked paprika. Cook for another 2 minutes.

  4. Add diced tomatoes and veggie broth. Bring to a boil.

  5. Reduce heat to low, cover, and simmer for 25-30 minutes until lentils are tender.

  6. Stir in spinach leaves and cook until wilted.

  7. For seasoning add salt and pepper to taste.

  8. Ladle stew into bowls, garnish with chopped cilantro, and serve warm.

3. **Tomato Basil Soup**
- Ingredients:
  - 1 tablespoon olive oil
  - 1 onion, chopped
  - 2 garlic cloves, minced
  - 1 can (28 oz) crushed tomatoes
  - 1 teaspoon dried basil
  - 1/2 teaspoon dried oregano
  - 4 cups low-sodium vegetable broth
  - Salt and pepper to taste
  - Chopped fresh basil leaves (for garnish)
  - Optional: 1/2 cup heavy cream or coconut milk for a creamy version

- Instructions:
  1. Heat the olive oil in a big pot over medium heat. Add the garlic and onion and sauté until tender.

  2. Add crushed tomatoes, dried basil, and dried oregano. Cook for 5 minutes, stirring occasionally.

  3. Add the veggie broth and heat until it boils.

  4. Reduce heat to low and simmer for 15-20 minutes to blend flavors.

  5. For seasoning add salt and pepper to taste.

  6. If desired, stir in heavy cream or coconut milk for a creamy texture.

7. Ladle soup into bowls, garnish with chopped fresh basil, and serve hot.

Additional Tips
- Meal Prep: Soups and stews often taste better the next day, making them ideal for meal prep and enjoyment throughout the week.

- Freezing: Many soups and stews freeze well, allowing for future quick and easy meals.

- Serve with Whole Grain Bread: Accompany soups and stews with whole grain bread or a side salad to round out the meal and add extra fiber.

Hearty soups and stews are versatile and nourishing lunch options that can be enjoyed throughout the year. Whether you prefer a comforting chicken and vegetable quinoa soup, a hearty lentil and vegetable stew, or a classic tomato basil soup, these recipes provide ample nutrients and flavors while supporting your health goals. By incorporating a variety of vegetables, lean proteins, and whole grains, you can create satisfying meals that keep you fueled and satisfied.

Nourishing Grain Bowls

Grain bowls are versatile, nutrient-packed meals that combine a base of wholesome grains with a variety of vegetables, proteins, and flavorful dressings. They are perfect for lunch, offering a balanced mix of macronutrients and micronutrients that align with the principles of the DASH (Dietary Approaches to Stop Hypertension) diet. Here's a guide to creating nourishing grain bowls:

Benefits of Nourishing Grain Bowls

1. Balanced Nutrition: Combines whole grains, lean proteins, healthy fats, and vegetables for a complete meal.

2. Customizable: Easily adjusted to suit personal preferences and dietary needs.

3. Convenient: Ideal for meal prepping and quick assembly.

Tips for Making Nourishing Grain Bowls

1. Choose Whole Grains: Use grains like quinoa, brown rice, farro, barley, or bulgur as the base for added fiber and nutrients.

2. Incorporate Lean Proteins: Add proteins such as grilled chicken, tofu, beans, lentils, or fish to support muscle health and satiety.

3. Add Fresh Vegetables: Include a variety of raw or cooked vegetables for color, texture, and vitamins.

4. Include Healthy Fats: Enhance flavor and nutrient absorption with healthy fats from sources like avocado, nuts, seeds, or olive oil.

5. Flavor with Dressings and Herbs: Use homemade dressings and fresh herbs to add flavor without excess sodium or unhealthy fats.

Nourishing Grain Bowl Recipes

1. **Mediterranean Quinoa Bowl**
- Ingredients:
  - 1 cup cooked quinoa
  - 1/2 cup cherry tomatoes, halved
  - 1/2 cucumber, diced
  - 1/4 cup Kalamata olives, sliced
  - 1/4 cup finely diced red onion
  - 1/4 cup feta cheese, crumbled
  - 1/4 cup hummus
  - Fresh parsley, chopped
  - A dressing of lemon juice and olive oil

- Instructions:
   1. In a bowl, layer cooked quinoa, cherry tomatoes, cucumber, olives, red onion, and feta cheese.
   2. Add a dollop of hummus on the side.
   3. Add a lemon juice and olive oil drizzle.
   4. Sprinkle with fresh parsley.
   5. Serve immediately and enjoy.

2. **Teriyaki Chicken Brown Rice Bowl**
- Ingredients:
  - 1 cup cooked brown rice
  - 1 grilled chicken breast, sliced
  - 1/2 cup steamed broccoli florets
  - 1/4 cup shredded carrots
  - 1/4 cup edamame beans
  - 1/4 cup sliced bell peppers
  - 2 tablespoons low-sodium teriyaki sauce
  - Sesame seeds for garnish
  - Green onions, sliced for garnish

- Instructions:
   1. In a bowl, layer cooked brown rice, sliced grilled chicken, steamed broccoli, shredded carrots, edamame, and bell peppers.
   2. Drizzle with teriyaki sauce.
   3. Sprinkle it with sesame seeds and green onions.
   4. Serve immediately and enjoy.

3. **Southwest Black Bean and Farro Bowl**
- Ingredients:
  - 1 cup cooked farro
  - 1/2 cup black beans, rinsed and drained
  - 1/2 cup corn kernels (fresh or frozen)
  - 1/2 avocado, diced
  - 1/2 cup cherry tomatoes, halved
  - 1/4 cup red onion, diced
  - Fresh cilantro, chopped
  - 1/4 cup salsa
  - Lime wedges for serving

- Instructions:
  1. In a bowl, layer cooked farro, black beans, corn, avocado, cherry tomatoes, and red onion.
  2. Add a spoonful of salsa on top.
  3. Sprinkle with fresh cilantro.
  4. Serve with lime wedges and enjoy.

Additional Tips
- Prep Ingredients Ahead: Cook grains and proteins in advance to make assembly quick and easy during busy weekdays.

- Mix and Match: Experiment with different grains, proteins, and vegetables to create new flavor combinations and keep meals exciting.

- Store Dressings Separately: If meal prepping, store dressings in separate containers to prevent grains and vegetables from becoming soggy.

Nourishing grain bowls are a versatile and convenient lunch option that provides a balanced mix of nutrients to support a healthy lifestyle. By incorporating whole grains, lean proteins, fresh vegetables, and healthy fats, you can create delicious and satisfying meals that align with the DASH diet principles. Whether you prefer a Mediterranean quinoa bowl, a teriyaki chicken brown rice bowl, or a Southwest black bean and farro bowl, these recipes offer a variety of flavors and nutrients that will keep you feeling full and energized all day.

Quick and Tasty Lunch Options

Finding time for a nutritious and delicious lunch can be challenging, especially on busy days. Quick and tasty lunch options can help you stay on track with your dietary goals without sacrificing flavor or nutrition. These recipes focus on simplicity, speed, and health, aligning with the principles of the DASH (Dietary Approaches to Stop Hypertension) diet.

Benefits of Quick and Tasty Lunch Options
1. Time-Efficient: Perfect for busy schedules, allowing you to prepare a wholesome meal in minimal time.

2. Nutritious: Combines essential nutrients to keep you energized and satisfied throughout the day.

3. Versatile: Offers flexibility in ingredients and preparation methods to suit personal preferences and available ingredients.

Tips for Making Quick and Tasty Lunches
1. Prep Ingredients Ahead: Pre-cut vegetables, cook proteins, and store grains to streamline meal assembly.

2. Use Simple Cooking Methods: Opt for no-cook, one-pan, or microwave-friendly recipes to save time.

3. Incorporate Balanced Nutrition: Ensure your meal includes a mix of carbohydrates, proteins, and healthy fats.

Quick and Tasty Lunch Recipes

1. **Greek Yogurt Chicken Salad**
- Ingredients:
  - 2 cups cooked chicken breast, shredded
  - 1/2 cup plain Greek yogurt
  - 1/4 cup mayonnaise (optional for creamy texture)
  - 1/2 cup celery, diced
  - 1/2 cup red grapes, halved
  - 1/4 cup finely diced red onion
  - 1/4 cup sliced almonds
  - 1 tablespoon lemon juice
  - Salt and pepper to taste
  - Whole grain bread, lettuce wraps, or whole grain crackers for serving

- Instructions:
  1. In a large bowl, combine shredded chicken, Greek yogurt, mayonnaise (if using), celery, grapes, red onion, sliced almonds, lemon juice, salt, and pepper.
  2. Mix well until all ingredients are evenly coated.
  3. Serve immediately on whole grain bread, lettuce wraps, or whole grain crackers.

2. **Veggie and Hummus Pita**
- Ingredients:
  - 1 whole grain pita pocket
  - 1/2 cup hummus (store-bought or homemade)
  - 1/4 cucumber, sliced
  - 1/4 red bell pepper, sliced
  - 1/4 cup shredded carrots
  - A handful of arugula or spinach leaves
  - 1/4 cup of feta cheese, crumbled (optional)

- Instructions:
  1. Cut the pita pocket in half and open each half to form pockets.
  2. Spread hummus inside each pita half.
  3. Fill with cucumber slices, red bell pepper, shredded carrots, and spinach or arugula leaves.
  4. Sprinkle with crumbled feta cheese if desired.
  5. Serve immediately.

3. **Tuna and Avocado Salad**
- Ingredients:
  - Five ounces (one can) of drained tuna

- 1/2 avocado, mashed
- 1 tablespoon Greek yogurt
- 1 tablespoon lemon juice
- 1 tablespoon chopped fresh parsley
- Salt and pepper to taste
- To serve, whole grain bread or lettuce wraps

- Instructions:
  1. In a medium bowl, combine tuna, mashed avocado, Greek yogurt, lemon juice, chopped parsley, salt, and pepper.
  2. Thoroughly stir until all items are incorporated.
  3. Serve immediately on whole grain bread or in lettuce wraps.

4. **Microwave Veggie Omelette**
- Ingredients:
  - 2 large eggs
  - 2 tablespoons milk (optional)
  - 1/4 cup diced bell peppers
  - 1/4 cup diced tomatoes
  - 1/4 cup chopped spinach
  - 1/4 cup shredded cheese (optional)
  - Salt and pepper to taste

- Instructions:
  1. In a microwave-safe bowl, whisk together eggs and milk (if using).
  2. Add diced bell peppers, tomatoes, spinach, salt, and pepper.
  3. Stir to combine.

4. Microwave on high for 1-2 minutes, stirring halfway through, until eggs are fully cooked.

5. Sprinkle with shredded cheese (if using) and microwave for an additional 15-30 seconds until cheese is melted.

6. Serve immediately.

5. **Quinoa and Black Bean Salad**
- Ingredients:
  - 1 cup cooked quinoa
  - 1/2 cup black beans, rinsed and drained
  - 1/2 cup corn kernels (fresh or frozen)
  - 1/2 cup cherry tomatoes, halved
  - 1/4 cup red onion, diced
  - 1/4 cup fresh cilantro, chopped
  - 2 tablespoons olive oil
  - 1 tablespoon lime juice
  - Salt and pepper to taste

- Instructions:

1. In a large bowl, combine cooked quinoa, black beans, corn, cherry tomatoes, red onion, and cilantro.

2. Drizzle with lime juice and olive oil.

3. Season with salt and pepper.

4. Toss well to combine.

5. Serve immediately or refrigerate for later.

Additional Tips

- Batch Cooking: Prepare larger quantities of recipes and store in the refrigerator for quick lunches throughout the week.

- Versatility: Use these recipes as a base and swap out ingredients based on what you have on hand or your preferences.

- Healthy Snacks: Pair your lunch with healthy snacks like fresh fruit, yogurt, or nuts to create a more complete meal.

Quick and tasty lunch options are essential for maintaining a healthy diet without compromising on time or flavor. By incorporating a variety of wholesome ingredients and simple preparation methods, you can create nutritious and delicious meals that support your dietary goals. Whether you choose a Greek yogurt chicken salad, a veggie and hummus pita, a tuna and avocado salad, a microwave veggie omelet, or a quinoa and black bean salad, these recipes offer a range of flavors and nutrients to keep you energized and satisfied throughout the day.

CHAPTER NINE

DINNER RECIPES

Balanced and Nutritious Main Dishes for Dinner

Dinner is an essential meal that helps replenish the body's nutrients after a long day and prepares it for the next. For those following the DASH (Dietary Approaches to Stop Hypertension) diet, dinner should be balanced, nutritious, and flavorful, aligning with dietary guidelines that focus on reducing sodium intake and including a lot of nutritious grains, lean proteins, fruits, and veggies.

Benefits of Balanced and Nutritious Dinner Dishes

1. Sustained Energy: Provides the necessary nutrients to support evening activities and restful sleep.

2. Nutrient-Dense: Offers a variety of vitamins, minerals, and antioxidants to support overall health.

3. Weight Management: Helps maintain a healthy weight by providing satisfying and low-calorie options.

Tips for Making Balanced and Nutritious Dinners

1. Incorporate Lean Proteins: Use sources like chicken, turkey, fish, tofu, beans, and legumes to build muscle and repair tissues.

2. Include Whole Grains: Choose whole grains like brown rice, quinoa, barley, or whole wheat pasta to add fiber and maintain satiety.

3. Add Plenty of Vegetables: Fill half your plate with a variety of colorful vegetables to increase vitamin, mineral, and fiber intake.

4. Healthy Fats: Incorporate healthy fats from sources like olive oil, avocados, nuts, and seeds for added flavor and heart health benefits.

5. Limit Sodium: Use herbs, spices, and natural flavor enhancers like lemon juice or vinegar instead of salt to reduce sodium intake.

Balanced and Nutritious Dinner Recipes

1. **Baked Lemon Herb Chicken with Quinoa and Roasted Vegetables**
- Ingredients:
  - 4 boneless, skinless chicken breasts
  - 2 tablespoons olive oil
  - Juice of 1 lemon
  - 2 teaspoons dried oregano
  - 1 teaspoon dried thyme
  - Salt and pepper to taste
  - 1 cup quinoa, rinsed
  - Two cups of low-sodium chicken broth or water
 - Two cups chopped mixed veggies (carrots, zucchini, bell peppers, etc.)
  - Fresh parsley, chopped (for garnish)

- Instructions:
  1. Set the oven's temperature to 400°F, or 200°C.
  2. In a small bowl, mix olive oil, lemon juice, oregano, thyme, salt, and pepper. Coat the chicken breasts with the mixture.
  3. Place chicken in a baking dish and bake for 25-30 minutes, or until cooked through.
  4. Meanwhile, in a medium pot, bring quinoa and water or chicken broth to a boil. Reduce heat to low, cover, and simmer for 15 minutes, or until quinoa is tender and water is absorbed.
  5. On a separate baking sheet, arrange mixed vegetables, drizzle with olive oil, and season with salt and pepper. Bake the veggies for 20 minutes, or until they are soft.

6. Serve chicken over quinoa with roasted vegetables on the side, garnished with fresh parsley.

2. **Salmon with Brown Rice and Steamed Broccoli**
- Ingredients:
  - 4 salmon filets
  - 2 tablespoons olive oil
  - Two teaspoons low-sodium soy sauce
  - 1 tablespoon honey
  - 2 cloves garlic, minced
  - 1 cup brown rice
  - 2 cups water
  - 4 cups broccoli florets
  - Lemon wedges (for serving)

- Instructions:
  1. Turn the oven on to 375°F, or 190°C.
  2. In a small bowl, mix olive oil, soy sauce, honey, and garlic. Brush the mixture over the salmon filets.
  3. Place salmon on a baking sheet lined with parchment paper and bake for 15-20 minutes, or until cooked through.
  4. Meanwhile, in a medium pot, bring brown rice and water to a boil. Reduce heat to low, cover, and simmer for 40-45 minutes, or until rice is tender and water is absorbed.
  5. In a steamer or microwave, steam broccoli florets until tender, about 5-7 minutes.
  6. Serve salmon over brown rice with steamed broccoli on the side, garnished with lemon wedges.

3. **Vegetarian Stuffed Peppers**
- Ingredients:
  - 4 bell peppers with the tops removed and the seeds extracted
  - 1 cup cooked quinoa
  - One can (15 ounces) of black beans, washed and drained
  - One cup of frozen or fresh corn kernels
  - 1/2 cup diced tomatoes
  - 1/2 cup shredded cheddar cheese (optional)
  - 1 teaspoon cumin
  - 1 teaspoon chili powder
  - Salt and pepper to taste
  - Fresh cilantro, chopped (for garnish)

- Instructions:
  1. Turn the oven on to 375°F, or 190°C.
  2. In a large bowl, combine cooked quinoa, black beans, corn, diced tomatoes, cumin, chili powder, salt, and pepper.
  3. Stuff each bell pepper with the quinoa mixture and place in a baking dish.
  4. If using, sprinkle shredded cheddar cheese on top of each stuffed pepper.
  5. Bake for 30 minutes with the foil covering. After removing the foil, roast the peppers for a further 10 minutes, or until they are soft.
  6. Serve immediately, garnished with fresh cilantro.

4. **Shrimp and Vegetable Stir-Fry with Brown Rice**
- Ingredients:
  - 1 pound large shrimp, peeled and deveined
  - 2 tablespoons olive oil
  - 2 cloves garlic, minced
  - 1 tablespoon ginger, minced
  - 1 red bell pepper, sliced
  - 1 yellow bell pepper, sliced
  - 1 cup snap peas
  - 2 cups broccoli florets
  - 3 tablespoons low-sodium soy sauce
  - 1 tablespoon rice vinegar
  - 1 tablespoon sesame oil
  - 2 cups cooked brown rice
  - Sesame seeds for garnish

- Instructions:
  1. In a large skillet or wok, heat olive oil over medium-high heat.
  2. Add garlic and ginger, sauté for 1 minute.
  3. Add shrimp and cook until pink, about 3-4 minutes. Remove shrimp and set aside.
  4. In the same skillet, add bell peppers, snap peas, and broccoli. Sauté for 5-7 minutes until vegetables are tender-crisp.
  5. Return shrimp to the skillet and add soy sauce, rice vinegar, and sesame oil. After combining everything, cook for a further two minutes.
  6. Serve stir-fry over cooked brown rice, garnished with sesame seeds.

5. **Tofu and Vegetable Curry**
- Ingredients:
  - 1 tablespoon olive oil
  - 1 onion, diced
  - 2 cloves garlic, minced
  - 1 tablespoon ginger, minced
  - 1 tablespoon curry powder
  - 1 can (14 oz) light coconut milk
  - One 14-oz can of chopped tomatoes
 - One cup of rinsed and drained chickpeas
 - Two cups chopped mixed veggies (carrots, zucchini, bell peppers, etc.)
 - One block (14 oz) of diced, firm tofu
  - Salt and pepper to taste
  - Fresh cilantro, chopped (for garnish)
  - Cooked brown rice or whole grain naan for serving

- Instructions:
  1. Heat the olive oil in a big pot over medium heat.
  2. Add onion, garlic, and ginger. Sauté until fragrant, about 2-3 minutes.
  3. Stir in curry powder and cook for 1 minute.
  4. Add coconut milk, diced tomatoes, chickpeas, and mixed vegetables. Bring to a simmer.
  5. Gently fold in cubed tofu and cook for 10-15 minutes, or until vegetables are tender and tofu is heated through.
  6. For seasoning add salt and pepper to taste.
  7. Serve curry over cooked brown rice or with whole grain naan, garnished with fresh cilantro.

Additional Tips

- Meal Prep: Prepare larger quantities of these dishes to enjoy as leftovers for lunch or dinner throughout the week.

- Freezing: Many of these dishes freeze well, making them convenient for future meals.

- Healthy Sides: Pair main dishes with healthy sides like a simple salad, steamed vegetables, or a light soup to create a well-rounded meal.

Balanced and nutritious main dishes for dinner are essential for maintaining a healthy lifestyle and supporting overall well-being. By incorporating lean proteins, whole grains, plenty of vegetables, and healthy fats, you can create delicious and satisfying meals that adhere to the principles of the DASH diet. Whether you choose baked lemon herb chicken with quinoa and roasted vegetables, salmon with brown rice and steamed broccoli, vegetarian stuffed peppers, shrimp and vegetable stir-fry, or tofu and vegetable curry, these recipes offer a variety of flavors and nutrients to keep you nourished and satisfied.

Flavorful Fish and Seafood Dishes for Dinner

Omega-3 fatty acids, vitamins, minerals, and lean protein can all be found in abundance in fish and seafood. Incorporating these into your dinner routine aligns well with the DASH (Dietary Approaches to Stop Hypertension) diet, which emphasizes heart-healthy eating. Fish and seafood dishes are versatile, quick to prepare, and can be flavored in numerous ways to keep meals exciting.

Benefits of Fish and Seafood

1. Heart Health: Rich in omega-3 fatty acids, which are known to support cardiovascular health.

2. High-Quality Protein: Provides essential amino acids necessary for muscle repair and overall health.

3. Nutrient-Dense: Packed with vitamins such as D and B2 (riboflavin), and minerals like calcium, phosphorus, iron, zinc, iodine, magnesium, and potassium.

4. Low in Saturated Fat: Offers a lean protein option with minimal saturated fat, making it a heart-healthy choice.

Tips for Cooking Fish and Seafood
1. Choose Fresh Ingredients: Opt for fresh or properly thawed seafood to ensure the best flavor and texture.

2. Season Simply: Use fresh herbs, citrus, garlic, and spices to enhance the natural flavors of the seafood without overwhelming them.

3. Cook Quickly: Most fish and seafood cook rapidly, making them ideal for quick dinners.

4. Watch the Temperature: Avoid overcooking, as this can result in a dry, tough texture. When fish flakes easily with a fork, it's done.

Flavorful Fish and Seafood Dinner Recipes

1. **Lemon Garlic Butter Shrimp**
- Ingredients:
  - 1 pound large shrimp, peeled and deveined
  - 3 tablespoons unsalted butter
  - 4 cloves garlic, minced
  - Juice of 1 lemon
  - Zest of 1 lemon
  - 2 tablespoons fresh parsley, chopped
  - Salt and pepper to taste
  - Lemon wedges for serving

- Instructions:
  1. Melt butter in a big skillet over medium-high heat.

2. Add garlic and sauté until fragrant, about 1 minute.

3. Add the shrimp and cook for 3–4 minutes on each side, or until they are pink and opaque.

4. Stir in lemon juice and zest, and season with salt and pepper.

5. Remove from heat and sprinkle with fresh parsley.

6. Serve immediately with lemon wedges.

2. **Baked Salmon with Dijon and Herb Crust**
- Ingredients:
  - 4 salmon filets
  - 2 tablespoons Dijon mustard
  - 2 tablespoons olive oil
  - 2 cloves garlic, minced
  - 1 tablespoon fresh dill, chopped
  - 1 tablespoon fresh parsley, chopped
  - 1 tablespoon fresh chives, chopped
  - Salt and pepper to taste
  - Lemon wedges for serving

- Instructions:
  1. Set the oven's temperature to 400°F, or 200°C.

  2. In a small bowl, mix Dijon mustard, olive oil, garlic, dill, parsley, chives, salt, and pepper.

  3. Place salmon filets on a baking sheet lined with parchment paper.

  4. Spread the Dijon herb mixture evenly over each filet.

  5. Bake the salmon for 12 to 15 minutes, or until it is well done and flake readily with a fork.

6. Serve immediately with lemon wedges.

3. **Mediterranean Grilled Swordfish**
- Ingredients:
  - 4 swordfish steaks
  - 3 tablespoons olive oil
  - Juice of 1 lemon
  - 2 cloves garlic, minced
  - 1 teaspoon dried oregano
  - 1 teaspoon dried thyme
  - Salt and pepper to taste
  - Fresh parsley, chopped (for garnish)

- Instructions:
  1. In a small bowl, mix olive oil, lemon juice, garlic, oregano, thyme, salt, and pepper.
  2. Place swordfish steaks in a shallow dish and pour the marinade over them. Marinate for at least 30 minutes.
  3. Turn the heat up to medium-high on the grill.
  4. Grill swordfish steaks for 4-5 minutes per side, or until cooked through and grill marks appear.
  5. Bake the fish for 15 to 20 minutes, or until it is cooked through and flakes readily with a fork.
  6. Serve immediately.

4. **Spicy Cajun Catfish**
- Ingredients:
  - 4 catfish filets
  - 2 tablespoons olive oil
  - 1 tablespoon Cajun seasoning
  - 1 teaspoon paprika

- 1 teaspoon garlic powder
- 1/2 teaspoon onion powder
- 1/2 teaspoon dried thyme
- 1/2 teaspoon dried oregano
- 1/4 teaspoon cayenne pepper (optional, for extra spice)
- Lemon wedges for serving

- Instructions:
  1. Turn the oven on to 375°F, or 190°C.
  2. In a small bowl, mix Cajun seasoning, paprika, garlic powder, onion powder, thyme, oregano, and cayenne pepper.
  3. Brush catfish filets with olive oil and sprinkle the seasoning mix evenly over both sides.
  4. Place catfish filets on a baking sheet lined with parchment paper.
  5. Bake the fish for 15 to 20 minutes, or until it is cooked through and flakes readily with a fork.
  6. Serve immediately with lemon wedges.

5. Thai Coconut Curry Fish

- Ingredients:
  - 1 pound white fish filets (such as cod, halibut, or tilapia)
  - 1 tablespoon olive oil
  - 1 onion, diced
  - 2 cloves garlic, minced
  - 1 tablespoon ginger, minced
  - 1 can (14 oz) light coconut milk
  - 2 tablespoons red curry paste
  - 1 tablespoon fish sauce

- 1 tablespoon lime juice
- 1 cup bell peppers, sliced
- 1 cup snap peas
- Fresh cilantro, chopped (for garnish)
- Lime wedges for serving

- Instructions:
1. Heat the olive oil in a big skillet over medium heat.
2. Add onion, garlic, and ginger. Sauté until fragrant, about 2-3 minutes.
3. Stir in coconut milk, red curry paste, and fish sauce. Bring to a simmer.
4. Add fish filets, bell peppers, and snap peas. Simmer for 10-12 minutes, or until fish is cooked through and vegetables are tender.
5. Stir in lime juice and remove from heat.
6. Serve immediately, garnished with fresh cilantro and lime wedges.

Additional Tips
- Pair with Healthy Sides: Serve fish and seafood dishes with sides like steamed vegetables, brown rice, quinoa, or a fresh salad to create a well-rounded meal.

- Experiment with Flavors: Try different herbs, spices, and marinades to keep meals interesting and flavorful.

- Cook in Batches: Prepare larger quantities of these dishes and store leftovers for quick and nutritious meals throughout the week.

Flavorful fish and seafood dishes are an excellent addition to any dinner routine, offering a combination of lean protein, healthy fats, and essential nutrients. By incorporating simple, fresh ingredients and a variety of cooking methods, you can create delicious and satisfying meals that align with the principles of the DASH diet. Whether you choose lemon garlic butter shrimp, baked salmon with Dijon and herb crust, Mediterranean grilled swordfish, spicy Cajun catfish, or Thai coconut curry fish, these recipes provide a range of flavors and nutrients to keep you nourished and satisfied.

Lean Poultry and Meat Dishes for Dinner

Lean poultry and meat are essential components of a balanced diet, providing high-quality protein, vitamins, and minerals necessary for overall health. When prepared in a healthy manner, these dishes can be both delicious and nutritious, fitting well into the DASH (Dietary Approaches to Stop Hypertension) diet. This guide offers comprehensive insights into creating lean poultry and meat dishes for dinner that are flavorful and adhere to DASH guidelines.

Benefits of Lean Poultry and Meat
1. High-Quality Protein: Essential for muscle repair, growth, and overall bodily functions.

2. Rich in Nutrients: Provides essential vitamins and minerals such as iron, zinc, and B vitamins.

3. Supports Satiety: Helps keep you full longer, aiding in weight management.

Tips for Cooking Lean Poultry and Meat

1. Choose Lean Cuts: Opt for skinless chicken breasts, turkey breasts, lean beef cuts (like sirloin or tenderloin), and pork tenderloin.

2. Trim Visible Fat: Remove any visible fat to reduce calorie and saturated fat intake.

3. Use Healthy Cooking Methods: Bake, grill, broil, or sauté instead of frying to maintain the nutritional integrity of the meat.

4. Season with Herbs and Spices: Use fresh herbs, spices, and natural flavorings instead of high-sodium seasonings.

Lean Poultry and Meat Dinner Recipes

1. Herb-Crusted Chicken Breast
- Ingredients:
  - 4 boneless, skinless chicken breasts

- 2 tablespoons olive oil
- 2 cloves garlic, minced
- 1 tablespoon fresh thyme, chopped
- 1 tablespoon fresh rosemary, chopped
- 1 tablespoon fresh parsley, chopped
- Salt and pepper to taste
- Lemon wedges for serving

- Instructions:
  1. Turn the oven on to 375°F, or 190°C.
  2. In a small bowl, mix olive oil, garlic, thyme, rosemary, parsley, salt, and pepper.
  3. Rub the herb mixture evenly over the chicken breasts.
  4. Place chicken on a baking sheet lined with parchment paper.
  5. Bake for 25-30 minutes, or until the chicken is cooked through and juices run clear.
  6. Serve immediately with lemon wedges.

2. Turkey Meatballs with Marinara Sauce
- Ingredients:
  - 1 pound ground turkey (93% lean)
  - 1/4 cup whole wheat breadcrumbs
  - 1/4 cup grated Parmesan cheese
  - 1 egg, beaten
  - 2 cloves garlic, minced
  - 1 tablespoon fresh basil, chopped
  - 1 tablespoon fresh parsley, chopped
  - Salt and pepper to taste
  - 2 cups low-sodium marinara sauce

- Whole grain pasta or zucchini noodles for serving

- Instructions:
   1. Turn the oven on to 375°F, or 190°C.
   2. In a large bowl, combine ground turkey, breadcrumbs, Parmesan cheese, egg, garlic, basil, parsley, salt, and pepper.
   3. Form the mixture into 1-inch meatballs and place on a baking sheet lined with parchment paper.
   4. Bake for 20-25 minutes, or until meatballs are cooked through and golden brown.
   5. In a large skillet, heat marinara sauce over medium heat. After ten minutes, add the meatballs and simmer.
   6. Serve meatballs and sauce over whole grain pasta or zucchini noodles.

3. **Balsamic Glazed Pork Tenderloin**
- Ingredients:
   - One pound or so of pork tenderloin
   - 2 tablespoons olive oil
   - 1/4 cup balsamic vinegar
   - 2 tablespoons honey
   - 2 cloves garlic, minced
   - 1 teaspoon dried thyme
   - Salt and pepper to taste

- Instructions:
   1. Set the oven's temperature to 400°F, or 200°C.

2. In a small bowl, mix balsamic vinegar, honey, garlic, thyme, salt, and pepper.

3. Place a large ovenproof skillet over medium-high heat with the olive oil. Add the pork tenderloin and fry it until it browns on all sides.

4. Pour balsamic glaze over the pork and transfer the skillet to the oven.

5. Roast for 20-25 minutes, or until the internal temperature reaches 145°F (63°C).

6. Let rest for 5 minutes before slicing and serving.

4. **Grilled Lemon Herb Turkey Cutlets**
- Ingredients:
  - 4 turkey cutlets
  - 3 tablespoons olive oil
  Zest and juice from one lemon
  - 2 cloves garlic, minced
  - 1 tablespoon fresh thyme, chopped
  - 1 tablespoon fresh rosemary, chopped
  - Salt and pepper to taste
  - Lemon wedges for serving

- Instructions:
  1. In a small bowl, mix olive oil, lemon juice, lemon zest, garlic, thyme, rosemary, salt, and pepper.
  2. Place turkey cutlets in a shallow dish and pour the marinade over them. Marinate for at least 30 minutes.
  3. Set the grill's temperature to medium-high.
  4. Grill turkey cutlets for 4-5 minutes per side, or until cooked through and grill marks appear.

5. Serve immediately with lemon wedges.

5. **Beef Stir-Fry with Vegetables**
- Ingredients:
  - 1 pound lean beef (such as sirloin or tenderloin), thinly sliced
  - 2 tablespoons olive oil
  - 2 cloves garlic, minced
  - 1 tablespoon fresh ginger, minced
  - 1 red bell pepper, sliced
  - 1 yellow bell pepper, sliced
  - 1 cup broccoli florets
  - 1 cup snap peas
  - 3 tablespoons low-sodium soy sauce
  - 1 tablespoon rice vinegar
  - 1 tablespoon sesame oil
  - Cooked brown rice for serving
  - Sesame seeds for garnish

- Instructions:
  1. In a large skillet or wok, heat olive oil over medium-high heat.
  2. Add garlic and ginger, sauté for 1 minute.
  3. Add sliced beef and cook until browned, about 4-5 minutes. Remove beef and set aside.
  4. In the same skillet, add bell peppers, broccoli, and snap peas. Sauté for 5-7 minutes until vegetables are tender-crisp.
  5. Return beef to the skillet and add soy sauce, rice vinegar, and sesame oil. After combining everything, cook for a further two minutes.

6. Serve stir-fry over cooked brown rice, garnished with sesame seeds.

Additional Tips
- Pair with Healthy Sides: Complement these dishes with sides like steamed vegetables, whole grains, or a fresh salad to create a balanced meal.

- Batch Cooking: Prepare larger quantities and store leftovers for quick, healthy meals throughout the week.

- Marinades and Rubs: Experiment with different marinades and spice rubs to keep flavors exciting and varied.

Lean poultry and meat dishes are integral to a balanced and nutritious dinner routine. By choosing lean cuts, using healthy cooking methods, and seasoning with fresh herbs and spices, you can create flavorful meals that adhere to the principles of the DASH diet. Whether you opt for herb-crusted chicken breast, turkey meatballs with marinara sauce, balsamic glazed pork tenderloin, grilled lemon herb turkey cutlets, or beef stir-fry with vegetables, these recipes provide a range of delicious and nutritious options to keep your dinners exciting and satisfying.

One-Pot and Sheet-Pan Dinners

One-pot and sheet-pan dinners are a game-changer for those seeking nutritious, delicious, and easy-to-prepare meals. These methods simplify cooking and cleanup, making them ideal for busy individuals and families. Perfectly suited for the DASH (Dietary Approaches to Stop Hypertension) diet, these dinners focus on using whole, fresh ingredients and balanced nutrition to support heart health and overall wellness. This guide offers insights into creating flavorful one-pot and sheet-pan dinners.

Benefits of One-Pot and Sheet-Pan Dinners

1. Convenience: Minimal preparation and cleanup, making them perfect for busy weeknights.

2. Balanced Nutrition: Easy to incorporate a variety of vegetables, lean proteins, and whole grains.

3. Flavorful: Cooking ingredients together enhances flavors, resulting in rich, delicious meals.

4. Versatility: Adaptable to various dietary preferences and seasonal ingredients.

Tips for Preparing One-Pot and Sheet-Pan Dinners

1. Choose High-Quality Ingredients: Fresh, whole ingredients yield the best flavor and nutrition.

2. Use Seasonings Wisely: Herbs, spices, and citrus zest enhance flavors without adding extra sodium.

3. Balance the Plate: Include a mix of lean proteins, vegetables, and whole grains or starchy vegetables.

4. Proper Cooking Techniques: Ensure even cooking by cutting ingredients into uniform sizes and preheating your oven or stovetop.

One-Pot Dinner Recipes

1. **One-Pot Chicken and Vegetable Stew**
- Ingredients:
  - 1 lb boneless, skinless chicken breasts, cut into bite-sized pieces
  - 2 tablespoons olive oil
  - 1 large onion, chopped
  - 2 cloves garlic, minced
  - 3 carrots, sliced
  - 2 celery stalks, sliced
  - 1 large potato, diced
  - 1 cup green beans, trimmed and cut into 1-inch pieces
  - 4 cups low-sodium chicken broth
  - 1 teaspoon dried thyme
  - 1 teaspoon dried rosemary
  - Salt and pepper to taste
  - 2 tablespoons fresh parsley, chopped (for garnish)

- Instructions:
   1. Heat the olive oil in a big pot over medium-high heat. After adding, sauté the chicken pieces until browned.
   2. Remove chicken and set aside. In the same pot, add onion and garlic, sauté until fragrant.
   3. Add carrots, celery, potato, and green beans. Cook for 5 minutes, stirring occasionally.
   4. Return chicken to the pot, pour in chicken broth, and add thyme and rosemary.
   5. Bring to a boil, then reduce heat and simmer for 20-25 minutes until vegetables are tender.
   6. Season with salt and pepper. Garnish with fresh parsley before serving.

2. One-Pot Vegetarian Chili
- Ingredients:
  - 2 tablespoons olive oil
  - 1 large onion, chopped
  - 2 cloves garlic, minced
  - 1 red bell pepper, chopped
  - 1 green bell pepper, chopped
  - 2 carrots, diced
  - 1 zucchini, diced
  - One can (15 ounces) of black beans, washed and drained
  - One can (15 oz) of rinsed and drained kidney beans
- One 15-oz can of chopped tomatoes
  - 2 cups vegetable broth
  - 2 tablespoons chili powder

- 1 teaspoon cumin
- 1 teaspoon smoked paprika
- Salt and pepper to taste
- One cup of frozen or fresh corn kernels
- Fresh cilantro, chopped (for garnish)
- Lime wedges (for serving)

- Instructions:
1. Heat the olive oil in a big pot over medium heat. Add the garlic and onion and sauté until tender.
2. Add bell peppers, carrots, and zucchini. Cook for 5-7 minutes, stirring occasionally.
3. Stir in black beans, kidney beans, diced tomatoes, vegetable broth, chili powder, cumin, and smoked paprika.
4. Bring to a boil, then simmer for 20 to 25 minutes on low heat.
5. Add corn kernels and cook for an additional 5 minutes.
6. Season with salt and pepper. Serve with lime wedges and garnish with fresh cilantro.

3. One-Pot Lemon Garlic Shrimp and Orzo
- Ingredients:
  - 2 tablespoons olive oil
  - One pound of shrimp with the peels removed
  - 4 cloves garlic, minced
  - 1 cup orzo
  - 2 cups low-sodium chicken broth
  - 1 cup cherry tomatoes, halved
  - 1 cup baby spinach
  - Zest and juice from one lemon

- 1/4 cup fresh parsley, chopped
- Salt and pepper to taste

- Instructions:
   1. In a big skillet over medium heat, warm up the olive oil. Add the shrimp and cook for 2 to 3 minutes on each side, or until pink. Remove and set aside.
   2. In the same skillet, add garlic and orzo. Cook for 1-2 minutes until fragrant.
   3. Add the chicken broth and heat it until it boils. Simmer for ten minutes over low heat, stirring now and then.
   4. Stir in cherry tomatoes and spinach. Cook until spinach is wilted.
   5. Return shrimp to the skillet and add lemon juice, zest, and fresh parsley.
   6. Season with salt and pepper. Serve immediately.

Sheet-Pan Dinner Recipes

1. **Sheet-Pan Roasted Chicken and Vegetables**
- Ingredients:
  - 4 boneless, skinless chicken thighs
  - 2 tablespoons olive oil
  - 2 cloves garlic, minced
  - 1 teaspoon dried thyme
  - 1 teaspoon dried rosemary
  - 1 large sweet potato, diced
  - 1 red bell pepper, sliced
  - 1 yellow bell pepper, sliced

- 1 red onion, sliced
- 1 zucchini, sliced
- Salt and pepper to taste
- Fresh parsley, chopped (for garnish)

- Instructions:
1. Preheat the oven to 400°F (200°C). Line a baking sheet with parchment paper.
2. In a small bowl, mix olive oil, garlic, thyme, rosemary, salt, and pepper.
3. Place chicken thighs on the baking sheet and brush with half of the olive oil mixture.
4. Arrange sweet potato, bell peppers, red onion, and zucchini around the chicken.
5. Drizzle the remaining olive oil mixture over the vegetables.
6. Roast for 25-30 minutes, until chicken is cooked through and vegetables are tender.
7. Add some fresh parsley as a garnish before serving.

2. **Sheet-Pan Salmon with Asparagus and Potatoes**
- Ingredients:
  - 4 salmon filets
  - 2 tablespoons olive oil
  - 2 cloves garlic, minced
  -Zest and juice from one lemon
  - 1 lb baby potatoes, halved
  - 1 bunch asparagus, trimmed
  - Salt and pepper to taste
  - Fresh dill, chopped (for garnish)

- Instructions:
  1. Preheat the oven to 400°F (200°C). Line a baking sheet with parchment paper.
  2. In a small bowl, mix olive oil, garlic, lemon juice, lemon zest, salt, and pepper.
  3. Place salmon filets on one side of the baking sheet and brush with the olive oil mixture.
  4. Arrange baby potatoes and asparagus on the other side of the baking sheet.
  5. Drizzle remaining olive oil mixture over the vegetables.
  6. Roast for 20-25 minutes, until salmon is cooked through and vegetables are tender.
  7. Before serving, garnish with fresh dill.

3. **Sheet-Pan Tofu and Vegetable Stir-Fry**
- Ingredients:
  - 1 block firm tofu, drained and cubed
  - 2 tablespoons olive oil
  - 2 cloves garlic, minced
  - 1 tablespoon soy sauce
  - 1 tablespoon rice vinegar
  - 1 red bell pepper, sliced
  - 1 yellow bell pepper, sliced
  - 1 cup broccoli florets
  - 1 cup snap peas
  - 1 teaspoon sesame oil
  - Sesame seeds (for garnish)
  - Cooked brown rice (for serving)

- Instructions:

1. Preheat the oven to 400°F (200°C). Line a baking sheet with parchment paper.

2. In a small bowl, mix olive oil, garlic, soy sauce, rice vinegar, and sesame oil.

3. Place tofu, bell peppers, broccoli, and snap peas on the baking sheet.

4. Drizzle with the olive oil mixture and toss to coat evenly.

5. Roast for 20-25 minutes, until tofu is golden brown and vegetables are tender.

6. Serve over cooked brown rice and garnish with sesame seeds.

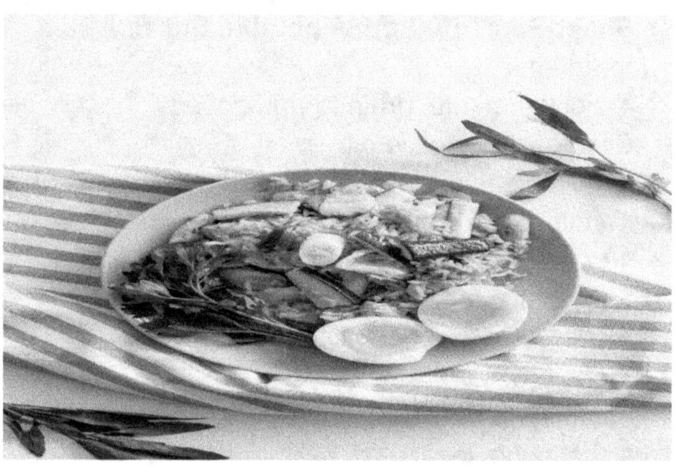

CHAPTER TEN

Snacks recipes

Healthy and Crunchy Snacks

Snacking can be a vital part of a balanced diet, especially when focusing on healthy and crunchy options. For those following the DASH (Dietary Approaches to Stop Hypertension) diet, it's important to choose snacks that not only satisfy cravings but also provide nutritional benefits. Healthy snacks can help maintain energy levels, curb overeating during meals, and offer essential nutrients. This guide will provide comprehensive insights into creating and enjoying healthy and crunchy snacks that align with the DASH diet principles.

Benefits of Healthy Snacking
1. Nutrient-Rich: Provides essential vitamins, minerals, and antioxidants.

2. Weight Management: Helps control hunger and prevents overeating during meals.

3. Steady Energy Levels: Maintains blood sugar levels and prevents energy crashes.

4. Heart Health: Reduces the intake of unhealthy fats and sodium, supporting cardiovascular health.

Tips for Healthy Snacking

1. Choose Whole Foods: Opt for whole, minimally processed foods such as fruits, vegetables, nuts, and seeds.

2. Watch Portions: Be mindful of portion sizes to avoid overeating, even with healthy snacks.

3. Balance Nutrients: Aim for a mix of protein, healthy fats, and fiber to keep you full and satisfied.

4. Prep Ahead: Prepare snacks in advance to ensure you have healthy options readily available.

Healthy and Crunchy Snack Ideas

1. **Fresh Vegetable Sticks with Hummus**
- Ingredients:
  - Carrot sticks
  - Celery sticks
  - Cucumber slices
  - Bell pepper strips
  - Cherry tomatoes
  - 1 cup hummus

- Instructions:
  1. Wash and cut vegetables into sticks or slices.
  2. Serve with a side of hummus for dipping.
  3. Remaining food should be refrigerated in an airtight container.

2. **Air-Popped Popcorn**
- Ingredients:
  - 1/4 cup popcorn kernels
  - 1 tablespoon olive oil (optional)
  - Salt and pepper to taste

- Instructions:
  1. Add the popcorn kernels to a big pot that has been heated to medium heat.
  2. Cover with a lid and shake the pot occasionally to prevent burning.
  3. Once popping slows, remove from heat and transfer to a bowl.
  4. Drizzle with olive oil (optional) and season with salt and pepper.

3. **Baked Kale Chips**
- Ingredients:
  - 1 bunch kale, washed and dried
  - 1 tablespoon olive oil
  - Salt and pepper to taste
  - 1 teaspoon garlic powder (optional)

- Instructions:
  1. Set the oven's temperature to 150°C/300°F.
  2. Tear kale leaves into bite-sized pieces, removing stems.
  3. Toss kale with olive oil, salt, pepper, and garlic powder (if using).
  4. Spread in a single layer on a baking sheet.
  5. Bake for 20-25 minutes, or until crispy, turning halfway through.

4. **Apple Slices with Nut Butter**
- Ingredients:
  - 1 large apple, sliced
  - Two teaspoons of peanut or almond butter

- Instructions:
  1. Wash and slice the apple.
  2. Serve apple slices with nut butter for dipping.
  3. Keep leftovers in the fridge in an airtight container.

5. **Greek Yogurt with Nuts and Berries**
- Ingredients:
  - 1 cup plain Greek yogurt
  1-/4 cup of mixed berries, including raspberries, strawberries, and blueberries
  - 2 tablespoons chopped nuts (almonds, walnuts, pecans)
  - 1 teaspoon honey (optional)

- Instructions:
  Pour Greek yogurt into a bowl using a spoon.
  2. Top with mixed berries and chopped nuts.
  3. Drizzle with honey (if using) and serve immediately.

6. **Roasted Chickpeas**
- Ingredients:
  - 1 can (15 oz) chickpeas, rinsed and drained
  - 1 tablespoon olive oil
  - 1 teaspoon smoked paprika

  - 1/2 teaspoon cumin
  - Salt and pepper to taste

- Instructions:
  1. Preheat the oven to 400°F (200°C).
  2. Use paper towels to pat the chickpeas dry.
  3. Toss chickpeas with olive oil, smoked paprika, cumin, salt, and pepper.
  4. Spread in a single layer on a baking sheet.
  5. Roast for 25-30 minutes, or until crispy, shaking the pan halfway through.

7. Whole Grain Crackers with Avocado
- Ingredients:
  - 1 avocado, mashed
  - 1 tablespoon lime juice
  - Salt and pepper to taste
  - Whole grain crackers

- Instructions:
  1. In a bowl, mash avocado with lime juice, salt, and pepper.
  2. Spread avocado mixture on whole grain crackers.
  3. Serve immediately.

8. Cucumber and Hummus Bites
- Ingredients:
  - 1 cucumber, sliced
  - 1 cup hummus
  - Paprika for garnish (optional)

- Instructions:
  1. Slice cucumber into rounds.
  2. Top each cucumber slice with a dollop of hummus.
  3. Sprinkle it with paprika (if using) and serve immediately.

9. **Trail Mix**
- Ingredients:
  - 1/4 cup almonds
  - 1/4 cup walnuts
  - 1/4 cup pumpkin seeds
  - 1/4 cup dried cranberries
  - 1/4 cup of optional dark chocolate chips

- Instructions:
  1. Mix all the ingredients inside a bowl.
 2. To make a quick and simple snack, store in an airtight container.

10. **Rice Cakes with Toppings**
- Ingredients:
  - Rice cakes
  - Toppings: avocado, tomato slices, cucumber slices, smoked salmon, cottage cheese

- Instructions:
  1. Choose your preferred toppings and arrange them on rice cakes.
  2. Serve immediately.

Additional Tips

- Seasonal Produce: Use seasonal fruits and vegetables to ensure freshness and variety.

- Hydration: Pair your snacks with water, herbal tea, or other low-sodium beverages to stay hydrated.

- Homemade Options: Making your own snacks allows you to control ingredients and avoid added sugars, salts, and unhealthy fats.

- Mindful Eating: Pay attention to your hunger and fullness cues to avoid mindless snacking.

Tasty Dips and Spreads

Dips and spreads are versatile additions to any meal, offering a flavorful and often nutrient-dense complement to vegetables, whole-grain crackers, and other DASH-friendly foods. For those adhering to the DASH (Dietary Approaches to Stop Hypertension) diet, incorporating healthy dips and spreads can enhance the enjoyment of snacks and sides while maintaining a focus on heart health. This guide will provide comprehensive insights into creating and enjoying a variety of tasty dips and spreads that align with DASH diet principles.

Benefits of Healthy Dips and Spreads
1. Nutrient Boost: Rich in vitamins, minerals, and healthy fats.

2. Flavor Enhancer: Adds taste and texture to otherwise plain snacks and sides.

3. Versatility: Can be paired with a wide range of foods, from vegetables to whole grains.

4. Heart Health: Low in unhealthy fats and sodium, supporting cardiovascular health.

Tips for Making Healthy Dips and Spreads

1. Use Fresh Ingredients: Opt for fresh herbs, vegetables, and fruits for maximum flavor and nutrition.

2. Balance Flavors: Combine savory, tangy, and sweet elements to create a well-rounded taste.

3. Control Portions: While healthy, some dips and spreads can be calorie-dense. Enjoy in moderation.

4. Minimize Added Salt: Use herbs and spices to enhance flavor without relying on salt.

Healthy and Tasty Dip and Spread Recipes

1. **Classic Hummus**
- Ingredients:
  - 1 can (15 oz) chickpeas, rinsed and drained
  - 1/4 cup tahini
  - 2 tablespoons olive oil
  - 2 tablespoons lemon juice
  - 2 cloves garlic, minced

- 1/2 teaspoon cumin
- Salt and pepper to taste
- Water, as needed

- Instructions:
  1. Toss everything together in a food processor.
  2. Blend until smooth, adding water as needed to reach desired consistency.
  3. Season with salt and pepper. Accompany with whole-grain crackers or vegetable sticks.

2. Avocado and Greek Yogurt Dip
- Ingredients:
  - 2 ripe avocados, peeled and pitted
  - 1/2 cup plain Greek yogurt
  - 2 tablespoons lime juice
  - 1 clove garlic, minced
  - Salt and pepper to taste
  - Fresh cilantro, chopped (for garnish)

- Instructions:
  1. In a bowl, mash avocados with Greek yogurt and lime juice.
  2. Stir in garlic, salt, and pepper.
  3. Garnish with fresh cilantro and serve with baked pita chips or raw vegetables.

3. Roasted Red Pepper and Feta Spread
- Ingredients:
  - Two roasted and peeled red bell peppers
  - 1/2 cup crumbled feta cheese
  - 2 tablespoons olive oil

- 1 tablespoon lemon juice
- 1 clove garlic, minced
- Salt and pepper to taste

- Instructions:
   1. Combine roasted peppers, feta, olive oil, lemon juice, and garlic in a food processor.
   2. Blend until smooth.
   3. Season with salt and pepper. Serve with whole-grain bread or crackers.

4. **Tzatziki**

- Ingredients:
   - 1 cup plain Greek yogurt
   - One shredded cucumber that has been pressed to remove extra water
   - 1 tablespoon lemon juice
   - 1 clove garlic, minced
   - 1 tablespoon fresh dill, chopped
   - Salt and pepper to taste

- Instructions:
   1. In a bowl, combine Greek yogurt, grated cucumber, lemon juice, garlic, and dill.
   2. Stir thoroughly and add pepper and salt to taste.
   3. Chill before serving. Serve with sliced vegetables or grilled meats.

5. **Black Bean Dip**
- Ingredients:
   - One can (15 ounces) of washed and drained black beans
   - 1/4 cup salsa
   - 1/4 cup plain Greek yogurt
   - 1 clove garlic, minced
   - 1 teaspoon cumin
   - Salt and pepper to taste
   - Fresh cilantro, chopped (for garnish)

- Instructions:
   1. Combine black beans, salsa, Greek yogurt, garlic, and cumin in a food processor.
   2. Blend until smooth.
   3. Season with salt and pepper. Garnish with fresh cilantro. Serve with baked tortilla chips or vegetable sticks.

6. **White Bean and Basil Dip**
- Ingredients:
   - One can (15 ounces) of washed and drained cannellini beans
   - 1/4 cup fresh basil leaves
   - 2 tablespoons olive oil
   - 2 tablespoons lemon juice
   - 1 clove garlic, minced
   - Salt and pepper to taste

- Instructions:
  1. Combine cannellini beans, basil, olive oil, lemon juice, and garlic in a food processor.
  2. Blend until smooth.
  3. Season with salt and pepper. Serve with whole-grain crackers or bread.

7. **Spicy Peanut Dip**
- Ingredients:
  - 1/2 cup natural peanut butter
  - 2 tablespoons soy sauce
  - 1 tablespoon rice vinegar
  - 1 tablespoon honey
  - 1 clove garlic, minced
  - 1 teaspoon grated ginger
  - 1/4 teaspoon (optional) red pepper flakes
  - Water, as needed

- Instructions:
  1. In a bowl, whisk together peanut butter, soy sauce, rice vinegar, honey, garlic, ginger, and red pepper flakes.
  2. Add water gradually to reach desired consistency.
  3. Serve with raw vegetables or rice paper rolls.

8. **Eggplant Dip (Baba Ganoush)**
- Ingredients:
  - 1 large eggplant
  - 2 tablespoons tahini
  - 2 tablespoons olive oil
  - 2 tablespoons lemon juice

- 2 cloves garlic, minced
- Salt and pepper to taste
- Fresh parsley, chopped (for garnish)

- Instructions:
  1. Preheat the oven to 400°F (200°C). Roast the eggplant until tender and the skin is charred, about 30-40 minutes.
  2. Let the eggplant cool, then peel and scoop out the flesh.
  3. In a food processor, combine eggplant flesh, tahini, olive oil, lemon juice, and garlic.
  4. Blend until smooth. Season with salt and pepper.
  5. Garnish with fresh parsley. Serve with vegetable sticks or pita bread.

9. **Herbed Cottage Cheese Spread**
- Ingredients:
  - 1 cup low-fat cottage cheese
  - 1 tablespoon fresh chives, chopped
  - 1 tablespoon fresh parsley, chopped
  - 1 tablespoon fresh dill, chopped
  - Salt and pepper to taste

- Instructions:
  1. In a bowl, mix cottage cheese with chives, parsley, and dill.
  2. Season with salt and pepper.
  3. Serve with whole-grain crackers or sliced vegetables.

10. **Sun-Dried Tomato and Basil Spread**
- Ingredients:
  - 1/2 cup chopped, drained, and sun-dried tomatoes in oil
  - 1/4 cup fresh basil leaves
  - 1/4 cup ricotta cheese
  - 2 tablespoons olive oil
  - 1 clove garlic, minced
  - Salt and pepper to taste

- Instructions:
  1. Combine sun-dried tomatoes, basil, ricotta, olive oil, and garlic in a food processor.
  2. Blend until smooth.
  3. Season with salt and pepper. Serve with whole-grain bread or crackers.

Additional Tips

- Storage: Most dips and spreads can be stored in an airtight container in the refrigerator for up to 5 days.

- Serving Ideas: Pair with fresh vegetable sticks, whole-grain crackers, or as a spread on sandwiches and wraps.

- Customizing Flavors: Experiment with different herbs, spices, and ingredients to create unique flavors that suit your taste preferences.

- Batch Preparation: Make larger batches and portion out servings for convenient snacking throughout the week.

Incorporating healthy and tasty dips and spreads into your diet can significantly enhance the enjoyment and nutritional value of snacks and sides. By focusing on fresh ingredients and balanced flavors, you can create a variety of dips and spreads that align with the DASH diet's goals of reducing blood pressure and promoting heart health. Whether you choose classic hummus, avocado and Greek yogurt dip, or roasted red pepper and feta spread, these recipes will add delicious and nutritious options to your snack repertoire.

Simple and Savory Sides

Sides are an integral part of a balanced meal, providing essential nutrients and complementing main dishes with flavors and textures. For those following the DASH (Dietary Approaches to Stop Hypertension) diet, incorporating simple and savory sides can enhance the overall dining experience while supporting heart health and nutritional goals. This guide will explore various simple and savory sides that are easy to prepare, delicious, and align with the DASH diet principles.

Importance of Savory Sides

1. Nutrient-Rich: Sides often include vegetables, grains, and legumes, offering vitamins, minerals, and fiber.

2. Balanced Meals: Adding sides to meals ensures a variety of food groups are included, promoting a balanced diet.

3. Flavor and Texture: Sides can introduce different flavors and textures, making meals more enjoyable and satisfying.

4. Heart Health: DASH-friendly sides are typically low in sodium and unhealthy fats, supporting cardiovascular health.

Tips for Preparing Savory Sides

1. Use Fresh Ingredients: Opt for fresh, seasonal produce for maximum flavor and nutritional benefits.

2. Minimize Salt: Enhance flavors with herbs, spices, and citrus instead of relying on salt.

3. Healthy Cooking Methods: Favor steaming, roasting, grilling, and sautéing over frying.

4. Batch Cooking: Prepare larger quantities and store leftovers for quick and easy meal additions.

Simple and Savory Side Recipes

1. **Garlic Roasted Vegetables**
- Ingredients:
  - 2 cups broccoli florets
  - 2 cups cauliflower florets
  - 1 red bell pepper, chopped
  - 1 yellow bell pepper, chopped
  - 2 tablespoons olive oil
  - 3 cloves garlic, minced
  - 1 teaspoon dried thyme
  - Salt and pepper to taste

- Instructions:
  1. Set the oven temperature to 425°F (220°C).
  2. In a large bowl, combine broccoli, cauliflower, bell peppers, olive oil, garlic, thyme, salt, and pepper.
  3. Arrange the vegetables on a baking sheet in a single layer.
  4. Roast for 25-30 minutes, or until vegetables are tender and slightly browned, stirring halfway through.

2. **Quinoa Pilaf**
- Ingredients:
  - 1 cup quinoa, rinsed
  - 2 cups low-sodium vegetable broth
  - 1 small onion, finely chopped
  - 1 carrot, diced
  - 1 celery stalk, diced
  - 1 tablespoon olive oil

- 1 teaspoon dried parsley
- Salt and pepper to taste

- Instructions:
  1. Heat the olive oil in a medium-sized pot over medium heat.
  2. Add onion, carrot, and celery. Sauté for approximately five minutes, or until veggies are soft.
  3. Stir in quinoa and cook for 1-2 minutes.
  4. Add vegetable broth, bring to a boil, then reduce heat to low and cover.
  5. Simmer for 15-20 minutes, or until quinoa is cooked and liquid is absorbed.
  6. Using a fork, fluff and season with parsley, salt, and pepper.

3. **Steamed Asparagus with Lemon**
- Ingredients:
  - 1 bunch asparagus, trimmed
  - 1 tablespoon olive oil
  - 1 tablespoon lemon juice
  - 1 teaspoon lemon zest
  - Salt and pepper to taste

- Instructions:
  1. Steam asparagus until tender but still crisp, about 3-5 minutes.
  2. In a small bowl, whisk together olive oil, lemon juice, lemon zest, salt, and pepper.
  3. Drizzle the lemon mixture over steamed asparagus and toss to coat.

4. **Sweet Potato Wedges**
- Ingredients:
  - Two big sweet potatoes, sliced into halves
  - 2 tablespoons olive oil
  - 1 teaspoon smoked paprika
  - 1/2 teaspoon garlic powder
  - Salt and pepper to taste

- Instructions:
  1. Preheat the oven to 400°F (200°C).
  2. In a large bowl, toss sweet potato wedges with olive oil, smoked paprika, garlic powder, salt, and pepper.
  3. Spread in a single layer on a baking sheet.
  4. Bake for 25-30 minutes, or until tender and slightly crispy, turning halfway through.

5. **Sautéed Green Beans with Almonds**
- Ingredients:
  - 1 pound green beans, trimmed
  - 2 tablespoons olive oil
  - 2 cloves garlic, minced
  - 1/4 cup sliced almonds
  - Salt and pepper to taste

- Instructions:
  1. Blanch green beans in boiling water for 2-3 minutes, then transfer to an ice bath to stop cooking.
  2. In a large skillet, warm the olive oil over medium heat.

3. Add the garlic and cook for approximately a minute, or until fragrant.

4. Add green beans and cook until heated through, about 5 minutes.

5. Stir in almonds and season with salt and pepper.

6. **Brown Rice and Vegetable Stir-Fry**
- Ingredients:
  - 1 cup brown rice, cooked
  - 1 red bell pepper, sliced
  - 1 yellow bell pepper, sliced
  - 1 small zucchini, sliced
  - 1 small yellow squash, sliced
  - 2 tablespoons olive oil
  - 2 tablespoons low-sodium soy sauce
  - 1 tablespoon sesame oil
  - 1 tablespoon sesame seeds
  - Salt and pepper to taste

- Instructions:
  1. Heat the olive oil in a big skillet over medium-high heat.
  2. Add bell peppers, zucchini, and yellow squash. Sauté for five to seven minutes, or until veggies are soft.
  3. Stir in cooked brown rice, soy sauce, and sesame oil.
  4. Cook for another 2-3 minutes, until heated through.
  5. Sprinkle with sesame seeds and season with salt and pepper.

7. **Cucumber and Tomato Salad**
- Ingredients:
  - 2 cups cherry tomatoes, halved
  - 1 large cucumber, diced
  - 1/4 red onion, thinly sliced
  - 2 tablespoons olive oil
  - 1 tablespoon red wine vinegar
  - 1 tablespoon fresh dill, chopped
  - Salt and pepper to taste

- Instructions:
  1. In a large bowl, combine cherry tomatoes, cucumber, and red onion.
  2. In a small bowl, whisk together olive oil, red wine vinegar, dill, salt, and pepper.
  3. Drizzle the veggies with the dressing and toss to coat.
  4. Serve immediately or chill before serving.

8. **Balsamic Glazed Carrots**
- Ingredients:
  - One pound of peeled and sliced sticks of carrots
  - 2 tablespoons olive oil
  - 2 tablespoons balsamic vinegar
  - 1 tablespoon honey
  - Salt and pepper to taste

- Instructions:
  1. Preheat the oven to 400°F (200°C).
  2. In a large bowl, toss carrots with olive oil, balsamic vinegar, honey, salt, and pepper.

3. Spread in a single layer on a baking sheet.

4. Roast for 20-25 minutes, or until carrots are tender and slightly caramelized, stirring halfway through.

9. **Spinach and Mushroom Sauté**

- Ingredients:
  - 2 tablespoons olive oil
  - 1 pound mushrooms, sliced
  - 2 cloves garlic, minced
  - 4 cups fresh spinach
  - Salt and pepper to taste

- Instructions:

1. Heat the olive oil in a big skillet over medium heat.

2. Add mushrooms and sauté until they release their moisture and start to brown, about 5-7 minutes.

3. Add the garlic and stir. Cook for approximately a minute, or until fragrant.

4. Add the spinach and simmer for 2 to 3 minutes, or until wilted.

5. Season with salt and pepper and serve immediately.

10. **Lemon Herb Couscous**

- Ingredients:
  - 1 cup whole-wheat couscous
  - 1 cup low-sodium vegetable broth
  - 1 tablespoon olive oil
  - 1 tablespoon lemon juice

- 1 teaspoon lemon zest
- 1 tablespoon fresh parsley, chopped
- 1 tablespoon fresh mint, chopped
- Salt and pepper to taste

- Instructions:
  1. Bring the vegetable broth to a boil in a medium-sized pot.
  2. Add the couscous, cover, and take the pan off the stove.
  3. Fluff couscous with a fork and stir in olive oil, lemon juice, lemon zest, parsley, and mint.
  4. For seasoning and salt and pepper to taste

Additional Tips

- Batch Cooking: Prepare larger quantities of sides and store leftovers for quick meal additions throughout the week.

- Serving Suggestions: Pair sides with lean proteins, whole grains, and a variety of vegetables for balanced meals.

- Seasonal Produce: Use seasonal vegetables and herbs to enhance flavor and nutritional value.

- Flavor Variations: Experiment with different herbs, spices, and cooking methods to create unique

and delicious sides.

Sweet Treats with a Healthy Twist

Indulging in sweet treats doesn't have to derail your health goals, especially when you're following the DASH (Dietary Approaches to Stop Hypertension) diet. By incorporating nutrient-dense ingredients and mindful preparation techniques, you can enjoy delicious and satisfying sweets that align with the DASH diet's principles. This guide will explore a variety of sweet treats with a healthy twist, ensuring you can satisfy your sweet tooth without compromising on health.

Importance of Healthy Sweet Treats
1. Nutrient-Rich: Using whole, unprocessed ingredients enhances the nutritional value.

2. Portion Control: Mindful portions prevent overindulgence and help maintain a balanced diet.

3. Reduced Added Sugars: Limiting added sugars supports heart health and overall well-being.

4. Flavorful and Satisfying: Healthy sweet treats can be just as delicious and satisfying as traditional desserts.

Tips for Making Healthy Sweet Treats
1. Use Natural Sweeteners: Opt for honey, maple syrup, dates, or ripe fruits instead of refined sugars.

2. Incorporate Whole Grains: Use whole wheat flour, oats, and other whole grains to increase fiber content.

3. Add Healthy Fats: Include nuts, seeds, and avocados for healthy fats that improve satiety.

4. Focus on Fresh Fruits: Utilize fresh fruits to add natural sweetness and nutrients.

Healthy Sweet Treat Recipes

1. **Chocolate Avocado Mousse**
- Ingredients:
  - 2 ripe avocados, peeled and pitted
  - 1/4 cup cocoa powder
  - 1/4 cup honey or maple syrup
  - 1/4 cup unsweetened almond milk
  - 1 teaspoon vanilla extract
  - Pinch of salt

- Instructions:
  1. Blend or process all ingredients in a food processor or blender.
  2. Blend until smooth and creamy.
  3. Before serving, place in the fridge for at least one hour.

2. **Berry Chia Pudding**
- Ingredients:
  - 1/4 cup chia seeds
  - 1 cup unsweetened almond milk

- One tablespoon of maple syrup or honey
- 1 teaspoon vanilla extract
- 1 cup mixed berries

- Instructions:
  1. In a bowl, whisk together chia seeds, almond milk, honey, and vanilla extract.
  2. Cover and refrigerate for at least 4 hours, or overnight, until thickened.
  3. Serve topped with mixed berries.

3. Baked Apple Slices
- Ingredients:
  - 4 apples, cored and sliced
  - 1 tablespoon coconut oil, melted
  - 1 teaspoon cinnamon
  - One tablespoon of maple syrup or honey

- Instructions:
  1. Preheat the oven to 350°F (175°C).
  2. In a bowl, toss apple slices with coconut oil, cinnamon, and honey.
  3. Arrange apple slices on a baking sheet.
  4. Bake for 20-25 minutes, or until tender and slightly caramelized.

4. Greek Yogurt and Fruit Parfait
- Ingredients:
  - 1 cup plain Greek yogurt
  - One tablespoon of maple syrup or honey
  - 1/2 cup granola (preferably low-sugar)

- 1 cup mixed fresh fruit (berries, banana slices, etc.)

- Instructions:
  1. In a bowl, mix Greek yogurt with honey.
  2. Layer yogurt, granola, and fresh fruit in a glass or bowl.
  3. Repeat layers and serve immediately.

5. Oatmeal Raisin Cookies
- Ingredients:
  - 1 cup rolled oats
  - 1/2 cup whole wheat flour
  - 1/2 teaspoon baking soda
  - 1/2 teaspoon cinnamon
  - 1/4 teaspoon salt
  - 1/4 cup coconut oil, melted
  - 1/4 cup honey or maple syrup
  - 1 egg
  - 1 teaspoon vanilla extract
  - 1/2 cup raisins

- Instructions:
  1. Preheat the oven to 350°F (175°C).
  2. In a bowl, mix oats, flour, baking soda, cinnamon, and salt.
  3. In another bowl, whisk together coconut oil, honey, egg, and vanilla extract.
  4. Combine wet and dry ingredients, then fold in raisins.
  5. Spoon dough onto a baking sheet in small amounts.

6. Bake for ten to twelve minutes, or until browned.

6. **Banana Nut Muffins**
- Ingredients:
  - 1 cup whole wheat flour
  - 1/2 cup rolled oats
  - 1 teaspoon baking powder
  - 1/2 teaspoon baking soda
  - 1/2 teaspoon cinnamon
  - 1/4 teaspoon salt
  - 2 ripe bananas, mashed
  - 1/4 cup honey or maple syrup
  - 1/4 cup unsweetened applesauce
  - 1 egg
  - 1 teaspoon vanilla extract
  - 1/2 cup chopped walnuts

- Instructions:
  1. Preheat the oven to 350°F (175°C).
  2. In a bowl, mix flour, oats, baking powder, baking soda, cinnamon, and salt.
  3. In another bowl, combine mashed bananas, honey, applesauce, egg, and vanilla extract.
  4. Combine the wet and dry ingredients, stirring just until blended.
  5. Fold in chopped walnuts.
  6. Divide batter into a muffin tin lined with paper liners.
  7. Bake for twenty-five to twenty-five minutes, or until a toothpick inserted in the center emerges clean.

7. Coconut Energy Balls

- Ingredients:
  - 1 cup rolled oats
  - 1/2 cup almond butter
  - 1/4 cup honey or maple syrup
  - 1/4 cup shredded coconut
  - 1/4 cup little chips made of dark chocolate
  - 1 teaspoon vanilla extract

- Instructions:
  1. Mix all the ingredients together inside a bowl.
  2. Mix until well combined.
  3. Roll mixture into small balls and refrigerate for at least 1 hour before serving.

8. Baked Pears with Walnuts and Honey

- Ingredients:
  - 2 pears, halved and cored
  - 1/4 cup chopped walnuts
  - 2 tablespoons honey
  - 1/2 teaspoon cinnamon

- Instructions:
  1. Preheat the oven to 350°F (175°C).
  2. Put the cut sides of the pear halves in a baking dish.
  3. Sprinkle it with chopped walnuts and cinnamon.
  4. Drizzle with honey.
  5. Bake for 20-25 minutes, or until the pears are tender.

9. **Frozen Yogurt Bark**
- Ingredients:
  - 2 cups plain Greek yogurt
  - A couple of teaspoons of honey or maple syrup
  - 1/2 cup mixed berries
  - 1/4 cup chopped nuts (almonds, pistachios, etc.)

- Instructions:
  1. Place parchment paper on a baking pan.
  2. In a bowl, mix Greek yogurt with honey.
  3. Spread yogurt mixture evenly on the baking sheet.
  4. Sprinkle with mixed berries and chopped nuts.
  5. Freeze until solid, or for at least two hours.
  6. Break into pieces and serve.

10. **Dark Chocolate-Dipped Strawberries**
- Ingredients:
  - 1 cup dark chocolate chips
  - 1 tablespoon coconut oil
  - 1 pint strawberries, washed and dried

- Instructions:
  1. In a microwave-safe bowl, combine dark chocolate chips and coconut oil.
  2. Microwave in 30-second intervals, stirring until melted and smooth.
  3. Dip strawberries into melted chocolate and place on a parchment-lined baking sheet.
  4. Refrigerate for at least 30 minutes, or until chocolate is set.

Additional Tips

- Portion Control: Enjoy sweet treats in moderation to maintain a balanced diet and avoid excessive calorie intake.

- Nutrient Density: Choose recipes that incorporate fruits, whole grains, nuts, and seeds to increase nutrient intake.

- Mindful Eating: Savor each bite and focus on the flavors and textures to enhance satisfaction and prevent overeating.

- Homemade vs. Store-Bought: Preparing treats at home allows you to control the ingredients and avoid unnecessary additives and sugars.

Sweet treats with a healthy twist can be a delightful and nutritious part of your diet, especially when following the DASH diet. By using whole, unprocessed ingredients and mindful preparation techniques, you can create delicious and satisfying desserts that support heart health and overall well-being.

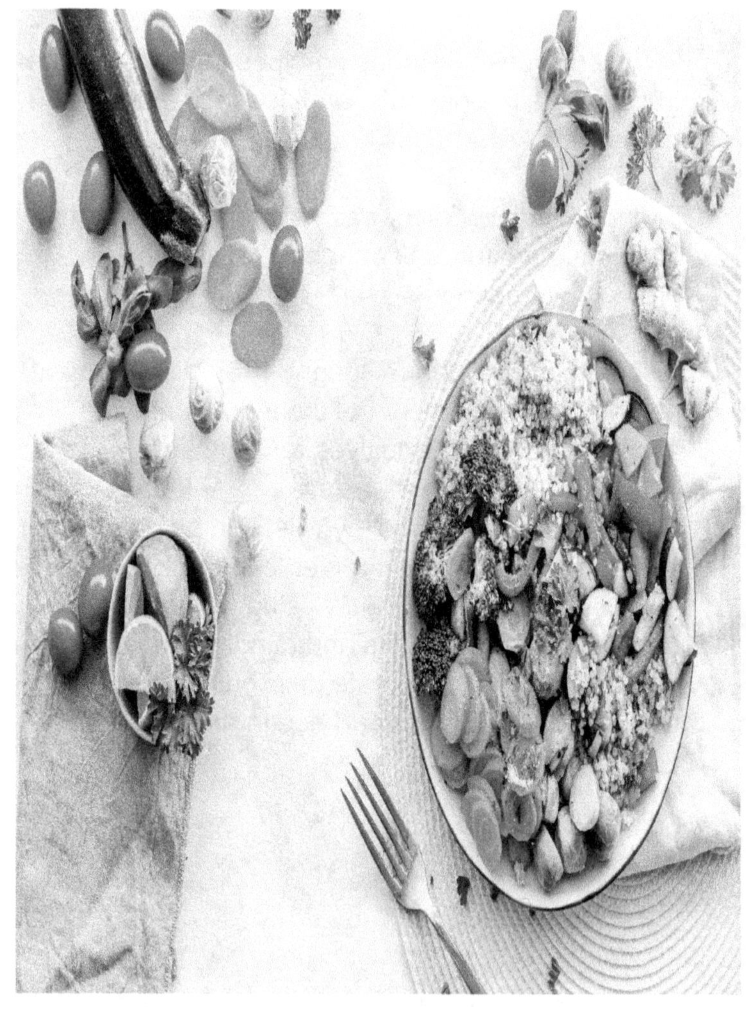

CHAPTER ELEVEN

Meal Planning and Prep

Meal planning and prep is a systematic approach to preparing and organizing meals ahead of time. It involves selecting recipes, shopping for ingredients, and cooking and storing meals in advance to streamline the process of eating healthy, balanced meals throughout the week. This approach is especially beneficial for those following specific dietary plans, like the DASH (Dietary Approaches to Stop Hypertension) diet, as it helps maintain consistency and adherence to nutritional goals. This guide will provide a comprehensive overview of meal planning and prep, its benefits, and practical tips for success.

The Importance of Meal Planning

Meal planning is a strategic approach to organizing and preparing meals ahead of time, which offers numerous benefits for individuals and families. It involves selecting recipes, making a grocery list, and prepping ingredients or complete meals in advance. This practice not only supports healthy eating habits but also contributes to better time management, financial savings, and reduced stress.

Health Benefits

1. Improved Nutrition:
   - Balanced Meals: Meal planning allows you to design nutritionally balanced meals, ensuring the inclusion of all essential food groups.
   - Portion Control: Preparing meals in advance helps control portion sizes, reducing the risk of overeating and maintaining a healthy weight.
   - Nutrient-Dense Foods: Planning encourages the use of whole, unprocessed foods, which are rich in vitamins, minerals, and antioxidants.

2. Consistent Healthy Eating:
   - Reduced Temptation: Having pre-prepared meals reduces the temptation to opt for unhealthy, convenience foods.
   - Dietary Adherence: For those following specific diets (e.g., DASH, vegetarian, gluten-free), meal planning ensures adherence to dietary guidelines.

3. Better Management of Dietary Restrictions:
   - Allergies and Intolerances: Meal planning helps manage food allergies and intolerances by allowing control over ingredients.
   - Chronic Conditions: Those with chronic conditions like diabetes or hypertension can better manage their health through tailored meal plans.

Financial Benefits

1. Cost Savings:
   - Reduced Impulse Buying: A well-thought-out grocery list based on a meal plan minimizes impulse purchases, saving money.
   - Bulk Buying: Planning ahead allows for bulk buying of staple items, which often reduces costs.

2. Decreased Food Waste:
   - Efficient Use of Ingredients: Meal planning ensures that all purchased ingredients are used efficiently, reducing food waste.
   - Leftover Management: Planning meals that incorporate leftovers prevents wastage and maximizes food utilization.

Time Management and Convenience

1. Time Savings:
   - Reduced Daily Cooking Time: Prepping meals in advance significantly reduces daily cooking time, allowing more time for other activities.
   - Streamlined Grocery Shopping: A detailed shopping list makes grocery trips quicker and more efficient.

2. Less Stress:
   - Eliminates Daily Decision Making: Knowing what you will eat each day reduces the stress of making meal decisions daily.

- Preparedness: Having meals ready to go provides peace of mind, especially during busy or unpredictable times.

Environmental Benefits

1. Lower Carbon Footprint:
   - Seasonal and Local Foods: Meal planning encourages the use of seasonal and locally sourced ingredients, which typically have a lower carbon footprint.
   - Reduced Packaging Waste: Buying in bulk and avoiding convenience foods reduces packaging waste, contributing to environmental sustainability.

2. Efficient Use of Resources:
   - Energy Savings: Cooking in batches uses less energy compared to cooking individual meals daily.
   - Water Conservation: Planning meals that use similar ingredients or cooking methods can reduce water usage in food preparation and clean-up.

Practical Tips for Effective Meal Planning

1. Start with a Weekly Plan:
   - Assess Your Schedule: Consider your weekly schedule, including work, social commitments, and family activities, to determine how many meals you need to prepare.

- Choose Recipes: Select a variety of recipes that are nutritious, easy to prepare, and suited to your dietary needs and preferences.

2. Create a Detailed Shopping List:
   - List by Categories: Organize your shopping list by categories (e.g., produce, dairy, grains) to make grocery shopping more efficient.
   - Include Staples: Ensure you have pantry staples (e.g., spices, oils, canned goods) on hand for quick meal preparation.

3. Prep Ingredients in Advance:
   - Batch Cooking: Prepare big quantities of veggies, grains, and proteins so they may be utilized for several meals a week.
   - Portion and Store: Portion meals into individual servings and store them in airtight containers to maintain freshness and convenience.

4. Stay Flexible:
   - Adjust as Needed: Be prepared to adjust your meal plan based on unexpected changes in your schedule or availability of ingredients.
   - Incorporate Leftovers: Plan meals that can easily incorporate leftovers, reducing waste and saving time.

5. Involve the Whole Family:
   - Family Preferences: Consider the preferences and dietary needs of all family members when planning meals.

- Cooking Together: Involve family members in meal prep to share responsibilities and enjoy quality time together.

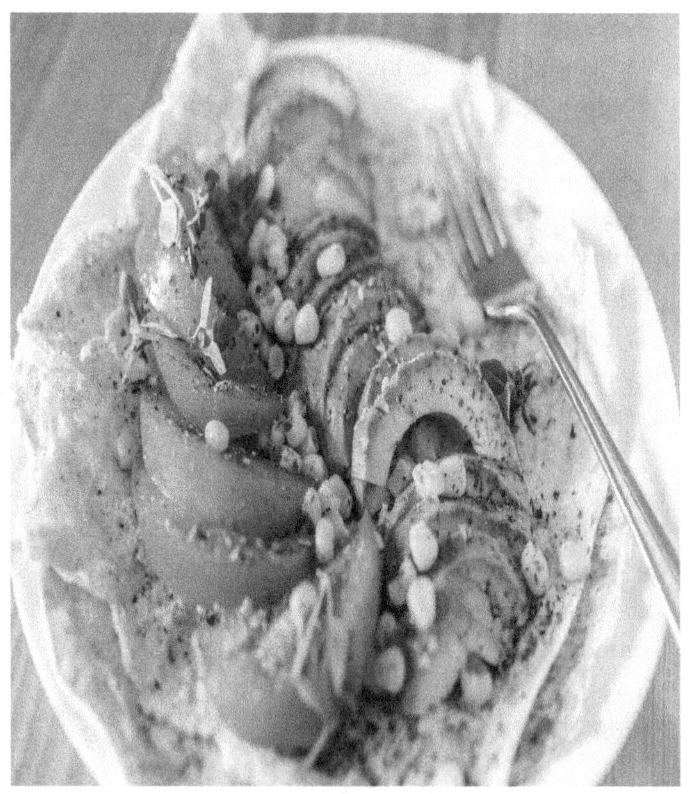

CHAPTER TWELVE

Creating a Weekly Meal Plan

Creating a weekly meal plan is a strategic process that involves organizing and preparing meals ahead of time. This approach not only supports healthier eating habits but also saves time, reduces stress, and can be more economical. Whether you're new to meal planning or looking to improve your current strategy, this guide provides a comprehensive overview of how to create an effective weekly meal plan.

Benefits of Weekly Meal Planning

1. Healthier Eating:
   - Balanced Diet: Ensures a balanced intake of essential nutrients by including a variety of food groups.
   - Portion Control: Helps manage portion sizes, which can aid in weight management and prevent overeating.

2. Time and Stress Management:
   - Efficiency: Reduces daily decision-making and cooking time, freeing up time for other activities.
   - Organization: Provides a clear plan for meals, reducing last-minute stress about what to cook.

3. Financial Savings:

- Budgeting: Allows for better budgeting and reduces the likelihood of eating out or ordering takeout.

- Reduced Waste: Minimizes food waste by using all purchased ingredients efficiently.

4. Improved Dietary Adherence:

- Consistency: Makes it easier to adhere to specific dietary requirements or goals, such as low-sodium diets, vegetarianism, or weight loss plans.

How to Plan Your Weekly Meals

1. Assess Your Week:

- Schedule: Review your weekly schedule to identify busy days when quick or pre-prepared meals might be needed.

- Meal Count: Determine how many breakfasts, lunches, dinners, and snacks you need to prepare.

2. Choose Recipes:

- Variety: Select a variety of recipes to ensure a balanced and interesting diet.

- Dietary Goals: Choose recipes that align with your dietary needs and preferences (e.g., DASH diet, vegetarian, low-carb).

- Seasonal Ingredients: Opt for seasonal and locally available ingredients for freshness and cost-effectiveness.

3. Create a Shopping List:
   - Categorize Items: Organize your shopping list
by sections of the grocery store (e.g., produce,
dairy, pantry items) to streamline the shopping
process.
   - Staples: Include pantry staples that you
frequently use to ensure you have a well-stocked
kitchen.

4. Prep and Cook:
   - Batch Cooking: Cook larger quantities of staple
items like grains, proteins, and roasted vegetables
that can be used in multiple meals.
   - Portioning: Divide meals into portions and store
them in airtight containers for easy access
throughout the week.
   - Prepping Ingredients: Wash, chop, and prep
ingredients in advance to save time during the
week.

5. Store and Label:
   - Storage: Use appropriate storage containers to
keep food fresh. Glass containers are great for
visibility and reheating, while freezer-safe
containers can preserve meals for longer periods.
   - Labeling: Label containers with the contents and
the date to keep track of freshness and meal
rotation.

6. Stay Flexible:

   - Adjustments: Be prepared to adjust your plan if unexpected events arise. Having a few versatile ingredients on hand can help you adapt quickly.

   - Leftovers: Incorporate leftovers into your meal plan to reduce waste and save time.

Tips for Meal Prep

Efficient meal prep is the cornerstone of maintaining a healthy diet, saving time, and reducing stress throughout the week. Whether you're a meal prep novice or a seasoned pro, these comprehensive tips will help streamline your process and make meal prepping a more manageable and enjoyable task.

Planning Phase

1. Set Clear Goals:

   - Determine your meal prep goals, whether it's for weight loss, muscle gain, saving money, or simply eating healthier. Having clear goals will guide your planning and prep efforts.

2. Create a Weekly Menu:

   - Make a weekly menu plan for breakfast, lunch, dinner, and snacks. Ensure your menu includes a variety of foods to meet your nutritional needs and keep things interesting.

3. Choose Simple Recipes:
   - Opt for recipes that are straightforward and require minimal ingredients and steps. This will make the prep process quicker and less overwhelming.

4. Balance Your Meals:
   - Ensure your planned meals have a good balance of protein, healthy fats, and carbohydrates. For vitamins, minerals, and fiber, make sure to eat an abundance of fruits and vegetables.

5. Use a Grocery List:
   - Create a thorough grocery list by using your meal plan as a guide. Organize it by sections of the store to save time and avoid unnecessary trips.

6. Consider Batch Cooking:
   - Choose recipes that can be cooked in large batches and stored for several days. Soups, stews, casseroles, and grain dishes are excellent options for batch cooking.

Shopping Phase

1. Shop Smart:
   - Follow your shopping list to prevent impulsive purchases. Shopping once a week will save time and help you avoid multiple trips to the store.

2. Buy in Bulk:
  - Purchase staple items like grains, beans, nuts, and frozen vegetables in bulk. This is often more cost-effective and ensures you have essential ingredients on hand.

3. Opt for Fresh and Seasonal:
  - Choose fresh, seasonal produce for better flavor and nutrition. Seasonal items are often cheaper and more readily available.

Preparation Phase

1. Organize Your Kitchen:
  - Before you start cooking, make sure your kitchen is clean and organized. Have all your tools, containers, and ingredients ready.

2. Invest in Quality Tools:
  - Good quality knives, cutting boards, pots, pans, and storage containers can make meal prep easier and more efficient.

3. Use Multi-Functional Appliances:
  - Appliances like slow cookers, Instant Pots, food processors, and blenders can significantly speed up meal prep.

4. Prepare Ingredients First:
  - Wash, chop, and prepare all your ingredients before you start cooking. This makes the cooking process smoother and faster.

5. Cook in Batches:
   - Cook multiple items at once. For example, roast vegetables while cooking grains on the stove and baking protein in the oven.

6. Multitask Efficiently:
   - While one dish is cooking, work on preparing another. This helps maximize your time in the kitchen.

Cooking Phase

1. Use Time-Saving Techniques:
   - Techniques like one-pot meals, sheet pan dinners, and slow cooker recipes can save a lot of time and reduce the number of dishes to clean.

2. Optimize Cooking Times:
   - Begin by cooking the foods that require the longest time. While they are cooking, work on shorter cooking items or prep work.

3. Flavor Enhancements:
   - Prepare and store spice mixes, sauces, and dressings in advance. This can quickly enhance the flavor of your meals.

Storage and Organization Phase

1. Choose the Right Containers:
   - Use airtight containers that are BPA-free and microwave safe. Glass containers are great for reheating, while plastic ones are lightweight and easy to store.

2. Label Everything:
   - Write the contents and the preparation date on the labels of your containers. This helps keep track of freshness and ensures you use older items first.

3. Portion Control:
   - Divide meals into individual portions. This makes it easier to grab a meal on the go and helps with portion control.

4. Store Smartly:
   - Store meals in the refrigerator for short-term use and in the freezer for longer-term storage. Ensure items are properly sealed to maintain freshness.

Reheating and Serving Phase

1. Safe Reheating:
   - Follow safe reheating practices to ensure food remains safe to eat. Reheat food to an internal temperature of 165°F (74°C).

2. Add Fresh Elements:
   - Enhance prepped meals with fresh elements like herbs, greens, or a squeeze of lemon juice before serving. This adds a fresh touch to your meal.

3. Flexible Meal Components:
   - Prep versatile components that can be mixed and matched throughout the week. For example, cooked chicken can be used in salads, wraps, and stir-fries.

Efficiency and Sustainability Tips

1. Use Leftovers Wisely:
   - Plan meals that can easily incorporate leftovers. For example, use leftover roasted vegetables in a frittata or a grain bowl.

2. Minimize Food Waste:
   - Be mindful of portion sizes and plan to use perishable items early in the week. Use vegetable scraps for making broths or composting.

3. Stay Organized:
   - Maintain organization in your freezer, fridge, and pantry. This helps you see what you have on hand and prevents food from getting lost and spoiling.

4. Evaluate and Adjust:
   - Evaluate what went well and poorly each week at the conclusion. Adjust your meal planning and prep strategies accordingly for better efficiency.

Sample Meal Prep Schedule

Saturday:
- Plan Meals: Decide on the meals for the upcoming week.
- Make a Grocery List: Based on the meal plan, create a detailed shopping list.

Sunday:
- Grocery Shopping: Purchase all the items on your list.
- Prepping Ingredients: Wash, chop, and prep ingredients.
- Cooking: Batch cooked proteins, grains, and vegetables. Prepare any sauces or dressings.
- Storage: Portion meals into containers and store in the refrigerator or freezer.

Throughout the Week:
- Reheat and Assemble: Reheat prepped components and assemble meals as needed.
- Adjust as Needed: Be flexible and adjust the plan if unexpected events arise.

CHAPTER THIRTEEN

Sample DASH Diet Meal Plans

The DASH (Dietary Approaches to Stop Hypertension) diet is designed to combat high blood pressure and promote overall heart health. It emphasizes the consumption of fruits, vegetables, whole grains, lean proteins, and low-fat dairy, while reducing the intake of sodium, added sugars, and unhealthy fats. Here are comprehensive sample meal plans for different calorie levels, offering a variety of nutritious and delicious options that adhere to the DASH diet guidelines.

1,200-Calorie DASH Diet Meal Plan

Day 1

- Breakfast:
  - Greek yogurt with fresh berries and a drizzle of honey
  - A slice of whole grain toast

- Morning Snack:
  - Apple slices with a tablespoon of almond butter

- Lunch:
  - Quinoa salad with mixed greens, cherry tomatoes, cucumber, chickpeas, and a lemon-tahini dressing

- Afternoon Snack:
  - Baby carrots and hummus

- Dinner:
  - Baked salmon served with a little sweet potato and steaming broccoli

Day 2

- Breakfast:
  - Overnight oats with chia seeds, sliced banana, and a sprinkle of cinnamon

- Morning Snack:
  - A handful of unsalted nuts

- Lunch:
  - Whole grain wrap with turkey, avocado, spinach, and a slice of tomato

- Afternoon Snack:
  - A small bowl of mixed berries

- Dinner:
  - Grilled chicken breast with quinoa and roasted Brussels sprouts

1,600-Calorie DASH Diet Meal Plan

Day 1

- Breakfast:
  - Smoothie with spinach, frozen mango, Greek yogurt, and a tablespoon of chia seeds

- Morning Snack:
  - Sliced cucumber with low-fat cottage cheese

- Lunch:
  - Lentil soup with a side of whole grain bread

- Afternoon Snack:
  - A small pear

- Dinner:
  - Grilled tofu with stir-fried vegetables (bell peppers, snap peas, carrots) and brown rice

Day 2

- Breakfast:
  - Poached egg and avocado on whole grain toast
  - A small orange

- Morning Snack:
  - Celery sticks with hummus

- Lunch:

  - Mixed greens salad with grilled chicken, cherry tomatoes, cucumbers, and balsamic vinaigrette

- Afternoon Snack:
  - Low-fat Greek yogurt with a handful of blueberries

- Dinner:
  - Baked cod with a side of quinoa and roasted asparagus

2,000-Calorie DASH Diet Meal Plan

Day 1

- Breakfast:
  - Eggs scrambled with mushrooms and spinach
  - A slice of whole grain toast with a small piece of fruit (like an apple)

- Morning Snack:
  - Greek yogurt with a tablespoon of flaxseeds and a handful of berries

- Lunch:
  - Whole grain pita stuffed with hummus, shredded carrots, cucumber slices, and grilled chicken

- Afternoon Snack:
  - A tiny bunch of almonds

- Dinner:

  - Grilled shrimp with a quinoa and vegetable
medley (zucchini, bell peppers, onions)
  - A side salad with mixed greens and balsamic
vinaigrette

Day 2

- Breakfast:
  - Smoothie bowl with blended frozen berries, a
banana, and almond milk, topped with granola and
chia seeds

- Morning Snack:
  - A small apple with peanut butter

- Lunch:
  - Whole grain pasta salad with cherry tomatoes,
black olives, feta cheese, and spinach, dressed
with olive oil and lemon juice

- Afternoon Snack:
  - Baby carrots with guacamole

- Dinner:
  - Lean beef stir-fry with mixed vegetables
(broccoli, bell peppers, carrots) served over brown
rice

2,400-Calorie DASH Diet Meal Plan

Day 1

- Breakfast:
  - Oatmeal made with low-fat milk, topped with sliced banana, walnuts, and a sprinkle of cinnamon

- Morning Snack:
  - A small bowl of mixed fruit (pineapple, berries, melon)

- Lunch:
  - Grilled chicken Caesar salad with romaine lettuce, cherry tomatoes, croutons, and a light Caesar dressing

- Afternoon Snack:
  - Pineapple chunks with low-fat cottage cheese

- Dinner:
  - Baked turkey meatballs with whole grain spaghetti and marinara sauce
  - Steamed green beans

Day 2

- Breakfast:
  - Smoothie with kale, pineapple, banana, Greek yogurt, and a tablespoon of flaxseeds

Morning Snack:
  - A small handful of trail mix (nuts, seeds, dried fruit)

- Lunch:
  - Whole grain wrap with grilled vegetables (zucchini, bell peppers, eggplant) and hummus

- Afternoon Snack:
  - Sliced bell peppers with tzatziki

- Dinner:
  - Grilled salmon with quinoa, roasted Brussels sprouts, and a mixed greens salad with a light vinaigrette

Tips for Following the DASH Diet

1. Focus on Fruits and Vegetables: Aim to fill half your plate with fruits and vegetables. They are rich in nutrients and fiber, which support heart health and overall wellness.

2. Choose Whole Grains: Opt for whole grains over refined grains. Whole grains provide more fiber and essential nutrients.

3. Include Lean Proteins: Incorporate lean protein sources such as fish, poultry, legumes, and low-fat dairy into your meals. These help build and repair tissues and support various bodily functions.

4. Limit Sodium Intake: Reduce sodium by choosing fresh foods over processed ones, using herbs and spices for flavor instead of salt, and reading food labels to select low-sodium options.

5. Watch Portion Sizes: Be mindful of portion sizes to avoid overeating. Portions can be better managed by using smaller bowls and plates.

6. Stay Hydrated: Drink plenty of water throughout the day. Choose water, herbal teas, or other low-calorie liquids in place of sugary drinks.

7. Plan and Prepare: Planning and preparing meals in advance can help ensure you stick to the DASH diet. Batch cooking and prepping ingredients can make it easier to prepare healthy meals during busy days.

By following these sample meal plans and tips, you can effectively implement the DASH diet into your daily routine, supporting your health and well-being.

Storing and Reheating Leftovers

Properly storing and reheating leftovers is essential to ensure food safety, maintain nutritional value, and enjoy the best possible taste and texture. This guide covers best practices for storing and reheating leftovers, including types of storage containers, labeling, refrigeration, freezing, and reheating techniques.

Storing Leftovers

1. Choose the Right Storage Containers

- Glass Containers: Ideal for both storing and reheating, as they do not retain odors or stains and are microwave-safe.
- Plastic Containers: Lightweight and convenient, but ensure they are BPA-free and safe for microwave use if you plan to reheat them.
- Vacuum-Sealed Bags: Great for freezing, as they remove air to prevent freezer burn and extend the shelf life of food.
- Mason Jars: Perfect for soups, stews, and salads, but avoid filling to the brim if freezing, as liquids expand when frozen.

2. Cool Food Before Storing

- Avoid Hot Storage: Allow hot food to cool slightly at room temperature (no more than 1-2 hours) before transferring to storage containers. This prevents condensation and bacterial growth.
- Shallow Containers: Use shallow containers to help food cool more quickly and evenly.

3. Label and Date

- Contents: Clearly label each container with the contents.

- Date: Include the date the food was prepared to keep track of freshness and ensure older items are consumed first.

4. Refrigeration

- Short-Term Storage: Refrigerate leftovers within 2 hours of cooking. Keep your refrigerator at or below 40°F (4°C).
- Shelf Life: Consume refrigerated leftovers within 3-4 days to ensure safety and quality.

5. Freezing

- Long-Term Storage: Freeze leftovers if you don't plan to eat them within a few days. Keep your freezer at or below 0°F (-18°C).
- Portion Control: Freeze leftovers in single-serving portions to make reheating easier and reduce waste.
- Avoid Overloading: Don't overcrowd the freezer, as proper air circulation is essential for maintaining a consistent temperature.

Reheating Leftovers

1. Safe Reheating Practices

- Internal Temperature: Reheat leftovers to an internal temperature of at least 165°F (74°C) to kill any potential bacteria. Use a food thermometer to check.

- Stirring and Rotating: Stir food or rotate containers
midway through reheating to ensure even heating.

2. Microwave Reheating

- Microwave-Safe Containers: Only use
microwave-safe containers and avoid plastic wraps
that may melt or release chemicals.
- Covering: Cover food with a microwave-safe lid or
microwave-safe plastic wrap to retain moisture and
prevent splatters.
- Power Setting: Use medium power settings to
prevent overcooking and drying out food.
- Standing Time: Let food stand for a minute or two
after microwaving to allow the heat to distribute
evenly.

3. Oven Reheating

- Low and Slow: Reheat food at a low temperature
(around 325°F or 165°C) to prevent drying out.
- Covering: Use aluminum foil to cover dishes and
retain moisture, especially for casseroles and
baked dishes.
- Stirring: Stir dishes like casseroles midway
through reheating for even temperature distribution.

4. Stovetop Reheating

- Sauces and Soups: Reheat sauces, soups, and
stews over medium heat, stirring frequently to
prevent sticking and ensure even heating.

- Pans and Skillets: Use a non-stick skillet to reheat items like rice, pasta, or stir-fries. Just a dash of broth or water will keep it from drying out.

5. Reheating Frozen Leftovers

- Thawing: For best results, thaw frozen leftovers in the refrigerator overnight before reheating. This lowers the possibility of bacterial growth and guarantees even heating.
- Microwave Thawing: If you need to thaw quickly, use the defrost setting on your microwave, but plan to cook the food immediately afterward.

Tips for Maintaining Quality and Safety

1. Avoid Refreezing: Do not refreeze leftovers that have been previously frozen and thawed, as this can degrade quality and increase the risk of bacterial growth.

2. Reheat Only Once: Reheat leftovers only once to minimize the risk of foodborne illness. If you have large portions, only reheat the amount you plan to consume.

3. Check for Spoilage: Always check for signs of spoilage before reheating leftovers. Discard food if it has an off smell, unusual texture, or visible mold.

4. Maintain Moisture: To prevent food from drying out, add a small amount of water, broth, or sauce before reheating. Covering dishes can also help retain moisture.

5. Even Heating: To ensure even heating, cut large pieces of food into smaller, uniform sizes. This is especially useful for meats and casseroles.

Properly storing and reheating leftovers is essential for maintaining food safety, quality, and taste. By following these comprehensive guidelines, you can enjoy nutritious, delicious meals with minimal waste and effort. Investing in the right storage containers, practicing safe cooling and reheating techniques, and maintaining an organized system for labeling and dating your leftovers will help you make the most of your meal prep efforts and keep your kitchen running smoothly.

CHAPTER FOURTEEN

Tips for Dining Out and Special Occasions on the DASH Diet

Staying committed to the DASH (Dietary Approaches to Stop Hypertension) diet can be challenging when dining out or attending special occasions. However, with some strategic planning and mindful choices, you can enjoy these experiences without compromising your dietary goals. This guide offers comprehensive tips to help you navigate restaurants, parties, and celebrations while adhering to the principles of the DASH diet.

Dining Out: General Strategies

1. Plan Ahead

- Research the Menu: Before heading out, check the restaurant's menu online. Look for dishes that align with the DASH diet, such as those featuring lean proteins, vegetables, and whole grains.
- Identify Healthy Options: Many restaurants offer lighter fare or heart-healthy sections. Choose items that are grilled, baked, steamed, or poached rather than fried or sautéed.

2. Be Specific with Your Order

- Customize Your Meal: Don't hesitate to ask for modifications. Request dressings and sauces on the side, opt for whole grain options, and ask for your dish to be prepared with minimal salt and butter.
- Portion Control: Restaurant portions can be large. Consider sharing a dish, ordering an appetizer as your main course, or asking for a to-go box at the beginning of your meal to save half for later.

3. Make Smart Choices

- Start with a Salad: Begin your meal with a green salad to fill up on fiber-rich vegetables. Choose a vinaigrette dressing on the side and use it sparingly.
- Select Lean Proteins: Opt for fish, chicken, or plant-based proteins. Avoid fatty cuts of meat and processed meats.
- Choose Whole Grains: If available, choose brown rice, quinoa, whole wheat pasta, or other whole grain options instead of refined grains.
- Load Up on Vegetables: Request extra vegetables as a side dish or as part of your main course. They are low in calories and high in nutrients.

4. Watch Your Sodium Intake

- Avoid High-Sodium Foods: Steer clear of dishes that are likely to be high in sodium, such as soups, sauces, pickles, and cured meats.
- Speak Up: Politely ask your server to inform the kitchen to use less salt in preparing your meal. Many restaurants are accustomed to accommodating dietary requests.

5. Beverages Matter

- Drink Water: Opt for water as your main beverage to stay hydrated and avoid extra calories from sugary drinks. Sparkling water with a slice of lemon or lime can be a refreshing alternative.
Control Alcohol Consumption: If you decide to drink, keep your intake to one drink for women and two for men each day.

Special Occasions: Parties and Celebrations

1. Prepare in Advance

- Eat a Healthy Snack: Before attending an event, eat a small, healthy snack such as a piece of fruit, yogurt, or a handful of nuts. By doing this, you can lessen your hunger and avoid overindulging.
- Bring a DASH-Friendly Dish: If it's a potluck or you're contributing to the meal, bring a dish that aligns with the DASH diet. This ensures you have at least one healthy option to enjoy.

2. Make Thoughtful Choices

- Survey the Options: Take a look at all the available foods before filling your plate. Choose a few healthy options and prioritize vegetables, lean proteins, and whole grains.
- Portion Control: Use a smaller plate if available, and avoid piling up your food. Start with moderate portions and go back for seconds only if you're still hungry.

3. Navigate Buffets Wisely

- Fill Up on Vegetables: Begin with salads and vegetable dishes to fill up on low-calorie, nutrient-dense foods.
- Limit High-Calorie Items: Be selective with richer, higher-calorie dishes. Choose small portions and savor each bite.
- Mind Your Sauces and Dressings: Use dressings and sauces sparingly. Opt for oil-based dressings or simple olive oil and vinegar.

4. Handle Desserts Smartly

- Small Portions: If you choose to indulge in dessert, take a small portion to satisfy your sweet tooth without overindulging.
- Healthier Options: Look for fruit-based desserts or those with less added sugar. Fresh fruit platters can be a refreshing and healthy choice.

5. Stay Active and Social

- Focus on Socializing: Engage in conversations and enjoy the company of others to take the focus off food.
- Incorporate Physical Activity: If possible, include some form of physical activity before or after the event, such as a walk or dancing.

Handling Peer Pressure and Temptations

1. Communicate Your Goals

- Be Honest: Let friends and family know about your commitment to the DASH diet. Most people will respect your choices and may even support you by offering healthier options.
- Decline Politely: If offered food that doesn't align with your diet, decline politely but firmly. You can say something like, "That looks delicious, but I'm trying to make healthier choices," or "No, thank you, I'm watching my sodium intake."

2. Practice Mindful Eating

- Eat Slowly: Savor each bite by taking your time. Eating slowly helps you enjoy your food more and gives your body time to signal when you're full.
- Listen to Your Body: Pay attention to your hunger and fullness cues. Eat until you're full, not until you're overstuffed.

Dining out and attending special occasions while following the DASH diet requires a combination of planning, smart choices, and mindful eating. By researching menus, making specific requests, and focusing on nutrient-dense foods, you can enjoy meals at restaurants and celebrations without compromising your dietary goals. Remember, the key is to make balanced choices that align with the principles of the DASH diet while still enjoying the social and culinary aspects of dining out and special occasions.

Making Healthy Choices at Restaurants
Eating out at restaurants can be an enjoyable experience, but it can also present challenges when you're trying to maintain a healthy diet like the DASH (Dietary Approaches to Stop Hypertension) diet. With some careful planning and mindful decisions, you can enjoy dining out while staying true to your nutritional goals. Here's a comprehensive guide to making healthy choices at restaurants.

1. **Do Your Homework**

Research the Menu Ahead of Time:
- Online Menus: Many restaurants post their menus online. Take a few minutes to review them and identify healthy options that align with the DASH diet.

- Nutritional Information: Some restaurants provide nutritional information on their websites. Use this data to make informed choices about calories, sodium, fats, and other nutrients.

Identify DASH-Friendly Restaurants:
- Cuisine Types: Some cuisines are more conducive to healthy eating than others. Look for restaurants that offer Mediterranean, Japanese, or other cuisines known for their healthy options.
- Special Requests: Choose restaurants that are willing to accommodate special dietary requests, such as low-sodium or low-fat preparations.

2. Be Mindful When Ordering

Ask for Modifications:
- Cooking Methods: Request that your food be grilled, baked, steamed, or poached instead of fried or sautéed in butter or oil.
- Sauces and Dressings: Ask for sauces and dressings on the side so you can control the amount you use. Opt for olive oil and vinegar over creamy dressings.
- Salt and Seasonings: Request your meal to be prepared with minimal salt. Ask for herbs, spices, lemon juice, or vinegar for added flavor.

Portion Control:
- Appetizers as Main Courses: Consider ordering an appetizer as your main course. Appetizers are

often smaller portions and can help you control your calorie intake.
- Sharing: Share a main dish with a friend or family member, or take half of your meal home. Many restaurant portions are significantly larger than what you need.

Choose Healthy Sides:
- Vegetables and Salads: Opt for vegetable sides or a side salad instead of fries or other high-calorie sides. Be mindful of dressings and toppings on salads.
- Whole Grains: Look for sides like brown rice, quinoa, or whole wheat bread.

3. Make Informed Choices

Healthy Starters:
- Salads: Start with a salad loaded with vegetables. Use dressings sparingly and avoid high-calorie toppings like croutons, bacon, and cheese.
- Soups: Choose broth-based soups over creamy ones. Vegetables, minestrone, or miso soup are good options.

Lean Proteins:
- Fish and Seafood: These are often lower in calories and saturated fats. Seek out baked, steaming, or grilled choices.
- Poultry: Choose skinless chicken or turkey. Avoid fried or breaded preparations.

- Plant-Based Proteins: Consider dishes featuring beans, lentils, tofu, or tempeh.

Healthy Fats:
- Nuts and Seeds: These can be a healthy addition to salads or dishes, but watch portion sizes as they are calorie-dense.
- Avocado: A good source of healthy fats, avocado can be a nutritious addition to your meal.

Carbohydrates:
- Whole Grains: Choose whole grains such as whole wheat bread, brown rice, or quinoa.
- Limit Refined Carbs: Avoid white bread, white rice, and other refined grains that lack fiber and nutrients.

4. Manage Sodium Intake

Identify High-Sodium Foods:
- Processed Foods: Avoid dishes that include processed meats, cheeses, pickles, and other high-sodium ingredients.
- Condiments and Sauces: Be cautious with soy sauce, ketchup, mustard, and other condiments that can be high in sodium.

Request Low-Sodium Options:
- Speak Up: Politely ask your server to have your meal prepared with less salt. Such demands are commonplace at many restaurants.

- Flavor Alternatives: Ask for herbs, spices, lemon juice, or vinegar to add flavor without extra sodium.

5. Beverages

Water First:
- Hydrate: Drinking water before and during your meal can help you stay hydrated and avoid mistaking thirst for hunger.
- Flavor It: If you prefer something with more taste, ask for sparkling water with a slice of lemon or lime.

Limit Sugary and Alcoholic Drinks:
- Skip the Sugary Drinks: Avoid sodas, sweetened teas, and other sugary beverages. They add empty calories and can spike your blood sugar.
- Moderate Alcohol: Use alcohol sparingly if you decide to consume it. Opt for a glass of wine or a light beer and avoid sugary cocktails.

6. Dessert

Healthier Sweet Options:
- Fruit-Based Desserts: Choose desserts that feature fresh fruit. These can be a satisfying way to end your meal without a lot of added sugar.
- Small Portions: If you decide to indulge in a richer dessert, consider sharing it or asking for a smaller portion.

Alternative Desserts:
- Yogurt Parfait: Some restaurants offer healthier dessert options like yogurt parfaits with fresh fruit and a drizzle of honey.
- Sorbet: Sorbet is often lower in calories and fat compared to ice cream or cakes.

7. Mindful Eating

Eat Slowly:
- Savor Your Food: Take your time to enjoy each bite. You can avoid overeating by eating slowly and learning to identify when you're full.
- Focus on Enjoyment: Pay attention to the flavors and textures of your food. Mindful eating enhances the dining experience and helps with portion control.

Listen to Your Body:
- Recognize Fullness: Stop eating when you feel satisfied, not stuffed. It's okay to leave food on your plate or take leftovers home.

CHAPTER FIFTEEN

DASH Diet-Friendly Fast Food Options

Navigating fast food options while adhering to the DASH (Dietary Approaches to Stop Hypertension) diet can be challenging due to the prevalence of high sodium, saturated fats, and added sugars in typical fast food fare. However, with careful choices and modifications, it is possible to find DASH-friendly options even at fast food restaurants. This guide provides comprehensive tips and suggestions to help you make healthier fast food choices that align with the principles of the DASH diet.

Understanding the DASH Diet

Before diving into specific fast food options, it's essential to understand the key principles of the DASH diet:

1. Emphasize Fruits and Vegetables: Aim for a variety of colorful fruits and vegetables.
2. Choose Whole Grains: Opt for whole grains over refined grains.
3. Include Lean Proteins: Focus on lean meats, poultry, fish, beans, and nuts.
4. Limit Sodium: Keep sodium intake low by avoiding high-sodium foods and condiments.

5. Reduce Saturated Fats and Added Sugars:
Choose foods low in saturated fats and avoid
sugary beverages and desserts.

General Tips for Fast Food Choices

1. Plan Ahead

- Review Menus Online: Many fast food chains
provide nutritional information on their websites.
Review these details beforehand to identify
healthier options.
- Look for Customization Options: Choose
restaurants that allow you to customize your order
to reduce sodium, fats, and calories.

2. Choose Smaller Portions

- Avoid Super-Sizing: Stick to regular or smaller
portion sizes to control calorie intake.
- Share Meals: Consider sharing a meal or side
with a friend to reduce portion size and caloric
intake.

3. Focus on Lean Proteins and Vegetables

- Grilled over Fried: Choose grilled chicken or fish
instead of fried versions.
- Add Vegetables: Opt for meals that include plenty
of vegetables or request extra veggies when
possible.

4. Beverages Matter

- Water First: Choose water or unsweetened beverages instead of sugary sodas or juices.
- Limit High-Calorie Drinks: Avoid milkshakes, flavored coffees, and other high-calorie beverages.

Specific Fast Food Options

1. Subway

Subway offers a variety of options that can be tailored to fit the DASH diet:

- Submarine Sandwiches: Choose a 6-inch whole grain sub. Opt for lean proteins like turkey breast, grilled chicken, or roast beef. Load up on vegetables like lettuce, tomatoes, cucumbers, peppers, and onions. Avoid high-sodium and high-fat condiments like mayo and opt for mustard or vinegar instead.
- Salads: Build a salad with plenty of vegetables and lean protein. Use olive oil and vinegar for dressing instead of creamy options.

2. McDonald's

While McDonald's is known for its burgers and fries, you can still find DASH-friendly choices:

- Grilled Chicken Sandwich: Order a grilled chicken sandwich without mayo or cheese. Opt for whole wheat buns if available.
- Salads: Choose a side salad with grilled chicken. Avoid high-fat dressings and croutons.
- Fruit and Yogurt Parfait: A lighter dessert option that includes fruit and low-fat yogurt.

3. Chipotle

Chipotle allows for a high degree of customization, making it easier to create a DASH-friendly meal:

- Bowl or Salad: Start with a salad base or a burrito bowl with brown rice. Choose black or pinto beans for added fiber and protein.
- Lean Proteins: Opt for grilled chicken, steak, or sofritas (tofu).
- Vegetables and Salsas: Load up on fajita vegetables, lettuce, and salsa. Avoid cheese, sour cream, and guacamole to keep calories and fats in check.
- Skip the Chips: Avoid adding chips to your meal, as they are high in sodium and calories.

4. Panera Bread

Panera Bread offers several healthy options that can fit the DASH diet:

- You Pick Two: Choose the "You Pick Two" option to combine a half sandwich, salad, or soup. Opt for whole grain bread and avoid high-sodium soups.
- Mediterranean Veggie Sandwich: This sandwich includes whole grain bread and plenty of vegetables. Ask for no feta cheese to reduce sodium.
- Salads: Select salads with plenty of vegetables and lean proteins. Use olive oil and vinegar for dressing.

5. Starbucks

Starbucks offers more than just coffee and pastries:

- Protein Boxes: Choose protein boxes that include fruit, vegetables, lean protein, and whole grain crackers.
- Salads and Bowls: Opt for salads and grain bowls with plenty of vegetables and lean proteins. Avoid high-fat dressings and toppings.
- Drinks: Choose plain coffee, tea, or unsweetened beverages. Avoid sugary syrups and whipped cream.

6. Taco Bell

Taco Bell can be surprisingly accommodating for DASH-friendly choices:

- Fresco Style: Order items "Fresco Style" to replace high-calorie sauces and cheese with fresh pico de gallo.
- Power Menu Bowl: Opt for the Power Menu Bowl with grilled chicken or steak. Customize by adding extra lettuce, tomatoes, and beans.
- Soft Tacos: Choose soft tacos with lean protein and ask for extra vegetables. Skip the cheese and creamy sauces.

Eating Well During Holidays and Celebrations

Maintaining a healthy diet, such as the DASH (Dietary Approaches to Stop Hypertension) diet, during holidays and celebrations can be challenging due to the abundance of rich foods, sugary treats, and indulgent meals. However, with mindful planning and smart choices, it is possible to enjoy festive occasions while staying true to your health goals. Here's a comprehensive guide to eating well during holidays and celebrations without sacrificing enjoyment.

1. **Plan Ahead**

Set Realistic Goals:
- Define Your Priorities: Decide what's most important to you during the celebration. Is it enjoying special foods, spending time with loved ones, or maintaining your health goals?
- Balance and Moderation: Aim for balance by enjoying your favorite holiday foods in moderation rather than deprivation.

Communicate Your Goals:
- Inform Hosts and Family: Let your hosts or family members know about your dietary preferences or restrictions. They may be able to accommodate your needs or provide healthier options.

2. **Make Smart Choices**

Focus on Nutrient-Dense Foods:
- Fill Up on Vegetables: Start your meal with a salad or load up on vegetable dishes. They are low in calories and high in fiber, vitamins, and minerals.
- Lean Proteins: Choose lean proteins such as turkey, chicken breast, fish, or legumes. These options provide essential nutrients without excess saturated fats.
- Whole Grains: Rather of refined grains, choose whole grains like brown rice, quinoa, or whole wheat bread.

Watch Portion Sizes:
- Use Small Plates: Using smaller plates can help control portion sizes and prevent overeating.
- Mindful Eating: Take your time, enjoy every bite, and be aware of your body's signals of hunger and fullness. Eat without stucking yourself beyond fullness.

3. **Navigate Festive Foods**

Holiday Dishes:
- Modify Recipes: Prepare traditional dishes with healthier substitutions, such as using low-fat dairy products, less salt, or reducing sugar content.
- Choose Wisely: Select dishes that align with the DASH diet principles, such as roasted vegetables, grilled meats, or steamed seafood.

Desserts and Sweets:
- Enjoy in Moderation: Indulge in small portions of your favorite desserts rather than multiple servings.
- Healthier Alternatives: Look for fruit-based desserts, like fruit salads or baked apples, which offer natural sweetness without added sugars.

4. **Stay Active**

Incorporate Physical Activity:
- Plan Activities: Organize outdoor games, walks, or activities that involve movement. Getting moving can help counteract the excess calories that are ingested during festivities.

- Stay Active Together: Invite friends and family to join you in physical activities to make it a fun and social event.

5. Hydration and Beverages

Drink Plenty of Water:
- Stay Hydrated: Drink water throughout the day to stay hydrated and maintain energy levels.
Control Alcohol: If you decide to consume alcohol, do so sparingly. Alternate alcoholic beverages with water to reduce overall calorie intake.

6. Manage Social Situations

Peer Pressure and Temptations:
- Be Assertive: Politely decline foods that don't align with your health goals. Something like, "No thank you, I'm trying to watch my sodium intake," might be appropriate.
- Offer to Bring a Dish: Bring a DASH-friendly dish to share with others. This guarantees that you will always have a healthy choice.

7. Practice Self-Care

Mindful Eating and Enjoyment:
- Focus on the Experience: Pay attention to the flavors and textures of the foods you eat. Mindful eating can enhance satisfaction and reduce overindulgence.

- Enjoy the Moment: Celebrate the occasion and the company of loved ones. Emphasize the social and cultural aspects of the gathering rather than just the food.

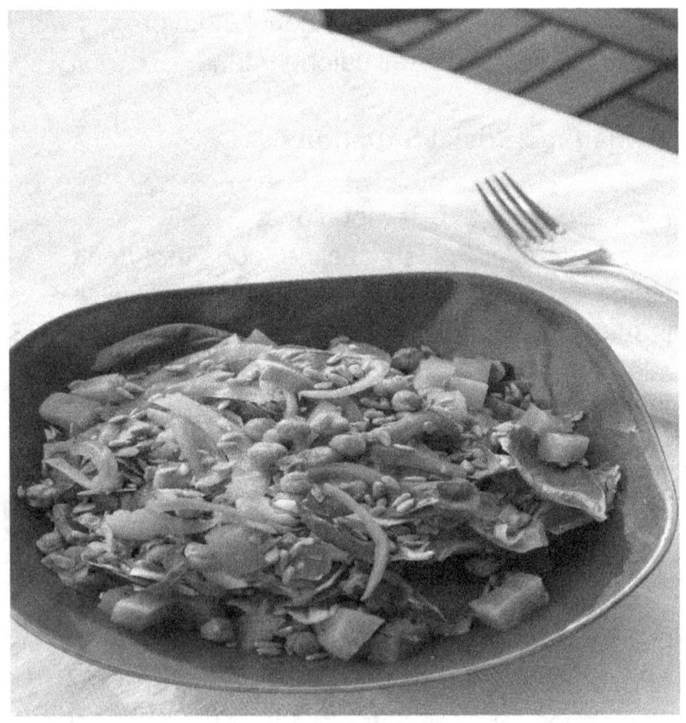

CHAPTER SIXTEEN

Overcoming challenges

Staying motivated and overcoming challenges while following a health-focused lifestyle such as the DASH (Dietary Approaches to Stop Hypertension) diet requires dedication, perseverance, and effective strategies. Whether you're aiming to manage hypertension or improve overall well-being, here's a comprehensive guide to help you stay motivated and conquer obstacles along the way:

1. Understanding Motivation

Identify Your Why:
- Health Goals: Clarify your reasons for following the DASH diet, such as reducing blood pressure, improving heart health, or achieving overall wellness.
- Personal Reasons: Reflect on how achieving these goals will positively impact your life, such as feeling more energetic, reducing medication dependency, or setting a good example for loved ones.

Set SMART Goals:
- Specific: Define clear and specific goals related to your health, diet, and lifestyle changes.
- Measurable: Establish measurable criteria to track your progress, such as daily servings of fruits and vegetables or weekly exercise sessions.
- Achievable: Make sure your goals are challenging but not impossible.
- Relevant: Ensure your goals align with your values and long-term health aspirations.
- Time-Bound: Assign deadlines or timelines to your goals to create accountability and motivation.

2. Strategies for Staying Motivated

Visualize Success:
- Create a Vision Board: Compile images, quotes, and goals related to your health journey to visualize your aspirations daily.
- Positive Affirmations: Use affirmations and positive self-talk to reinforce your commitment and resilience.

Celebrate Milestones:
- Acknowledge Achievements: Celebrate small victories, such as reaching a weight loss milestone, consistently meeting your daily fruit and vegetable intake, or reducing sodium intake.

Find Support:
- Build a Support Network: Surround yourself with supportive individuals, such as friends, family

members, or online communities, who share your
health goals and can offer encouragement.
- Accountability Partner: Partner with someone who
can hold you accountable for your actions and
provide motivation during challenging times.

3. **Overcoming Challenges**

Identify Triggers and Obstacles:
- Recognize Challenges: Identify common barriers
to sticking with the DASH diet, such as cravings for
unhealthy foods, social pressure, time constraints,
or stress.

Develop Coping Strategies:
- Problem-Solving Skills: Develop strategies to
address challenges proactively, such as meal
planning, stress management techniques (like yoga
or meditation), or finding alternative ways to
socialize without focusing on food.
- Healthy Substitutions: Discover healthier
alternatives to your favorite foods, such as
swapping high-sodium snacks for fresh fruits or
replacing sugary drinks with infused water.

Learn from Setbacks:
- Resilience: View setbacks as opportunities for
learning and growth rather than reasons to give up.
Reflect on what triggered the setback and
strategize ways to prevent similar situations in the
future.

4. **Maintain Variety and Enjoyment**

Explore New Recipes:
- Cooking Adventures: Experiment with new DASH-friendly recipes to keep meals exciting and flavorful.
- Cuisine Exploration: Discover international cuisines that align with the DASH diet principles, adding variety to your meal plan.

Mindful Eating:
- Savor Meals: Practice mindful eating by paying attention to flavors, textures, and sensations while eating. This can reduce overindulgence and increase contentment.

5. **Seek Professional Guidance**

Consult Healthcare Providers:
- Nutritional Counseling: Schedule appointments with registered dietitians or healthcare providers who specialize in hypertension management and can provide personalized guidance.
- Medical Support: Discuss any challenges or concerns related to your health journey with your healthcare team for tailored advice and support.

DASH diet shopping list

Creating a comprehensive DASH (Dietary Approaches to Stop Hypertension) diet shopping list is essential for stocking your kitchen with nutritious foods that align with the principles of the diet. The DASH diet emphasizes consuming foods rich in nutrients such as potassium, calcium, magnesium, fiber, and low in sodium. Here's a detailed guide to help you build a DASH diet shopping list:

1. **Fruits and Vegetables**

Fresh Produce:
- Leafy Greens: collard greens, spinach, kale, Swiss chard, and lettuce
- Colorful Vegetables: Bell peppers, carrots, tomatoes, cucumbers, broccoli, cauliflower
- Berries: Blueberries, strawberries, raspberries, blackberries
- Citrus Fruits: Oranges, grapefruits, lemons, limes
- Bananas and Apples: Great for snacks and adding to breakfasts

Frozen Options:
- Frozen Berries: Convenient for smoothies and desserts
- Mixed Vegetables: Such as stir-fry mixes or broccoli-cauliflower blends

2. **Whole Grains**

- Brown Rice: Rich in fiber and nutrients, suitable for main dishes and side dishes
- Quinoa: High in protein and fiber, versatile for salads, side dishes, or as a base for bowls
- Whole Wheat Pasta: Use in pasta dishes with tomato-based sauces or vegetables
- Oats: Ideal for breakfast porridge, overnight oats, or adding to smoothies

3. **Lean Proteins**

- Chicken Breast: Skinless and boneless, suitable for grilling, baking, or stir-frying
- Turkey Breast: Lean cuts for sandwiches, wraps, or salads
- Fish: Salmon, trout, tuna, or other fatty fish rich in omega-3s
- Beans and Legumes: Black beans, chickpeas, lentils, kidney beans for vegetarian protein sources

4. **Dairy and Alternatives**

- Low-Fat Milk: Opt for skim or 1% milk for calcium and vitamin D
- Greek Yogurt: Low-fat or fat-free varieties, plain or lightly sweetened
- Cheese: Low-fat options such as feta, mozzarella, or cottage cheese

- Plant-Based Milks: Unsweetened almond milk,
soy milk, or oat milk fortified with calcium and
vitamin D

5. **Nuts, Seeds, and Healthy Fats**

- Almonds, Walnuts, Pistachios: Rich in
heart-healthy fats, great for snacks or adding to
salads
- Chia Seeds, Flaxseeds: High in omega-3 fatty
acids and fiber, sprinkle on yogurt or oatmeal
- Avocados: Versatile for salads, sandwiches,
wraps, or as a topping for toast

6. **Herbs, Spices, and Condiments**

- Herbs: Fresh herbs like basil, cilantro, parsley,
and dried herbs like oregano, thyme, and rosemary
for flavoring dishes
- Spices: Cinnamon, turmeric, cumin, paprika, garlic
powder, and chili powder for adding flavor without
added sodium
- Condiments: Olive oil, balsamic vinegar, mustard,
low-sodium soy sauce, salsa, and tomato paste for
cooking and seasoning

7. **Pantry Staples**

- Canned Beans: Low-sodium varieties of black
beans, kidney beans, chickpeas for convenience
- Canned Tomatoes: Diced tomatoes, tomato
sauce, or paste for soups, stews, and sauces

- Whole Grain Bread: Choose varieties with at least 3 grams of fiber per serving for sandwiches or toast
- Low-Sodium Broth: Vegetable, chicken, or beef broth for soups and cooking grains

8. Beverages

- Water: Drink lots of water to stay hydrated throughout the day.
- Green Tea: Rich in antioxidants, a healthy alternative to sugary beverages

9. Snacks and Treats

- Dark Chocolate: Opt for varieties with at least 70% cocoa for a healthier treat
- Popcorn: Air-popped or lightly seasoned popcorn for a low-calorie snack option

10. Miscellaneous

- Eggs: Versatile for breakfast, salads, sandwiches, or as a protein source in main dishes
- Honey or Maple Syrup: Natural sweeteners for adding to yogurt, oatmeal, or homemade dressings
- Nutritional Yeast: Adds a cheesy flavor and nutrients to dishes, great for vegan recipes

Tips for Shopping:

- Read Labels: Choose products with lower sodium content and minimal added sugars.

- Shop the Perimeter: Focus on fresh produce, lean proteins, dairy, and avoid heavily processed foods.
- Plan Meals: Create a meal plan based on your shopping list to minimize waste and ensure you have ingredients for balanced meals throughout the week.

By using this comprehensive DASH diet shopping list as a guide, you can stock your kitchen with nutrient-dense foods that support heart health, lower blood pressure, and promote overall well-being. Adjust quantities based on your household size and individual dietary needs to maintain consistency in following the DASH diet principles.

CONCLUSION

In conclusion, embarking on a journey with the DASH (Dietary Approaches to Stop Hypertension) diet offers not just a path to better health but a sustainable lifestyle filled with flavorful and nourishing meals. As we've explored throughout this Simple DASH Diet Cookbook for Beginners, the principles of the DASH diet emphasize wholesome ingredients, balanced nutrition, and thoughtful meal planning. By incorporating a variety of fruits, vegetables, whole grains, lean proteins, and healthy fats into your daily meals, you not only support your cardiovascular health but also enhance overall well-being.

Throughout this cookbook, we've provided you with essential tools, from understanding the science behind the DASH diet to practical tips for grocery shopping, meal preparation, and enjoying delicious recipes that align with these principles. Whether you're starting your day with energizing smoothies, savoring wholesome oatmeal, enjoying vibrant salads for lunch, or indulging in nutritious dinners, each recipe is crafted to support your health goals while satisfying your taste buds.

As you continue on your DASH diet journey, remember that small, consistent steps lead to significant changes. Celebrate each milestone, whether it's trying a new recipe, mastering a cooking technique, or noticing improvements in your health markers. Stay motivated by nurturing a supportive environment and embracing the joy of preparing and sharing nourishing meals with loved ones.

Ultimately, adopting the DASH diet isn't just about what you eat; it's about embracing a lifestyle that prioritizes health, wellness, and longevity. By making informed food choices and incorporating regular physical activity, you're investing in your future well-being. Let this cookbook serve as your guide and inspiration as you navigate the path to a healthier, happier you through the principles of the DASH diet. Cheers to your journey to better health!